VOLUME **3**

Curriculum
Beginning

RECOMMENDED CITATIONS

AEPS®-3

Bricker, D., Dionne, C., Grisham, J., Johnson, J. J., Macy, M., Slentz, K., & Waddell, M. (2022). *Assessment, Evaluation, and Programming System for Infants and Children, Third Edition (AEPS®-3)*. Brookes Publishing Co.

Volume 1 AEPS®-3 User's Guide

Bricker, D., & Johnson, J. J. (Eds.). (2022). *AEPS®-3 Volume 1: User's guide.* In D. Bricker, C. Dionne, J. Grisham, J. J. Johnson, M. Macy, K. Slentz, & M. Waddell, *Assessment, Evaluation, and Programming System for Infants and Children, Third Edition (AEPS®-3)*. Brookes Publishing Co.

Volume 2 AEPS®-3 Assessment

Bricker, D., & Johnson, J. J. (Eds.). (2022). *AEPS®-3 Volume 2: Assessment.* In D. Bricker, C. Dionne, J. Grisham, J. J. Johnson, M. Macy, K. Slentz, & M. Waddell, *Assessment, Evaluation, and Programming System for Infants and Children, Third Edition (AEPS®-3)*. Brookes Publishing Co.

Volume 3 AEPS®-3 Curriculum–Beginning

Grisham, J., & Slentz, K. (Eds.). (2022). *AEPS®-3 Volume 3: Curriculum—Beginning.* In D. Bricker, C. Dionne, J. Grisham, J. J. Johnson, M. Macy, K. Slentz, & M. Waddell, *Assessment, Evaluation, and Programming System for Infants and Children, Third Edition (AEPS®-3)*. Brookes Publishing Co.

Volume 4 AEPS®-3 Curriculum–Growing

Grisham, J., & Slentz, K. (Eds.). (2022). *AEPS®-3 Volume 4: Curriculum—Growing.* In D. Bricker, C. Dionne, J. Grisham, J. J. Johnson, M. Macy, K. Slentz, & M. Waddell, *Assessment, Evaluation, and Programming System for Infants and Children, Third Edition (AEPS®-3)*. Brookes Publishing Co.

Volume 5 AEPS®-3 Curriculum–Ready

Grisham, J., & Slentz, K. (Eds.). (2022). *AEPS®-3 Volume 5: Curriculum—Ready.* In D. Bricker, C. Dionne, J. Grisham, J. J. Johnson, M. Macy, K. Slentz, & M. Waddell, *Assessment, Evaluation, and Programming System for Infants and Children, Third Edition (AEPS®-3)*. Brookes Publishing Co.

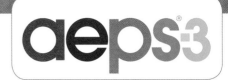

VOLUME 3

Curriculum
Beginning

edited by

Jennifer Grisham, Ed.D.
University of Kentucky
Lexington

and

Kristine Slentz, Ph.D.
Western Washington University
Bellingham

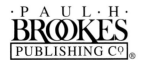
·P A U L ·H·
BROOKES
PUBLISHING C^O®

Baltimore • London • Sydney

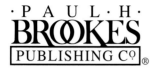

Paul H. Brookes Publishing Co.
Post Office Box 10624
Baltimore, Maryland 21285-0624
USA

www.brookespublishing.com

Typeset by Progressive Publishing Services, York, Pennsylvania.
Manufactured in the United States of America by Sheridan Books, Inc.

All examples in this book are composites. Any similarity to actual individuals or circumstances is coincidental, and no implications should be inferred.

To order, contact Brookes Publishing Co. or visit www.brookespublishing.com.

Please see Recommended Citations at the beginning of this book for a list of AEPS-3 volumes. Printable masters of the AEPS-3 forms are also available. All AEPS-3 materials are available from Brookes Publishing Co., P.O. Box 10624, Baltimore, Maryland 21285-0624 (800-638-3775 or 410-337-9580).

To find out more about AEPS-3, please visit www.aepsinteractive.com.

Library of Congress Cataloging-in-Publication Data

Names: Bricker, Diane D., editor. | Johnson, JoAnn, editor. | Grisham, Jennifer, editor. |
    Slentz, Kristine, editor.
Title: Assessment, evaluation, and programming system for infants and children / edited by
    Diane Bricker, JoAnn (JJ) Johnson.
Other titles: At head of title: AEPS-3
Description: Third edition. | Baltimore, Maryland: Paul H. Brookes Publishing Co., [2022] |
    Includes bibliographical references and index.
Contents: v. 1. User's guide / edited by Diane Bricker, JoAnn (JJ) Johnson—v. 2. Assessment / edited by
    Diane Bricker, JoAnn (JJ) Johnson—v. 3. Curriculum-beginning / edited by Jennifer Grisham and
    Kristine Slentz—v. 4. Curriculum-growing / edited by Jennifer Grisham and Kristine Slentz—v. 5.
    Curriculum-ready edited by Jennifer Grisham and Kristine Slentz.
Identifiers: LCCN 2021022790| ISBN 9781681255194 (v. 1; paperback) | ISBN 9781681255200
    (v. 2; paperback) | ISBN 9781681255217 (v. 3; paperback) | ISBN 9781681255224 (v. 4; paperback) |
    ISBN 9781681255231 (v. 5; paperback)
Subjects: LCSH: Assessment, Evaluation, and Programming System. | Child development—Testing. |
    Child development deviations—Diagnosis.
Classification: LCC RJ51.D48 A87 2022 | DDC 618.92/0075—dc23
LC record available at https://lccn.loc.gov/2021022790

British Library Cataloguing in Publication data are available from the British Library.

2025   2024   2023   2022   2021

10   9   8   7   6   5   4   3   2   1

Contents

About the Authors

Diane Bricker, Ph.D., Professor Emerita and Former Director, Early Intervention Program, Center on Human Development, and Former Associate Dean for Academic Programs, College of Education, University of Oregon, Eugene

Dr. Bricker served as Director of the Early Intervention Program at the Center on Human Development, University of Oregon, from 1978 to 2004. She was a professor of special education, focusing on the fields of early intervention and social communication.

Her professional interests have addressed three major areas: early intervention service delivery approaches, curriculum-based assessment and evaluation, and developmental-behavioral screening. Dr. Bricker's work in early intervention approaches has been summarized in two volumes: *An Activity-Based Approach to Early Intervention, Fourth Edition* (with J. Johnson & N. Rahn; Brookes Publishing Co., 2015), and *An Activity-Based Approach to Developing Young Children's Social Emotional Competence* (with J. Squires; Brookes Publishing Co., 2007). Her work in curriculum-based assessment and evaluation has focused on the development of the *Assessment, Evaluation, and Programming System for Infants and Children* (*AEPS*®; Brookes Publishing Co., 1993, 1996, 2002, 2022). This measure and associated curricula provide intervention personnel with a system for the comprehensive assessment of young children with results that link directly to curricular content and subsequent evaluation of child progress.

Dr. Bricker has been a primary author of the *Ages & Stages Questionnaires*® (*ASQ*®; with J. Squires; Brookes Publishing Co., 1995, 1999, 2009) and has directed research activities on the ASQ system starting in 1980. *Developmental Screening in Your Community: An Integrated Approach for Connecting Children with Services* (with M. Macy, J. Squires, & K. Marks; Brookes Publishing Co., 2013) offers a comprehensive system for creating and operating communitywide developmental-behavioral screening programs for young children.

Dr. Bricker's distinctions include the Division of Early Childhood, Council for Exceptional Children Service to the Field Award, December 1992, and the Peabody College Distinguished Alumna Award, May 1995.

Carmen Dionne, Ph.D., Chairholder, United Nations Educational, Scientific and Cultural Organization (UNESCO), and Lecturer, Department of Psychoeducation, University of Québec at Trois-Rivières (UQTR), Canada

Dr. Dionne is Professor of Special Education at the University of Québec at Trois-Rivières (UQTR), where she has worked since 1997. She led the Canada Research Chair in Early Intervention from 2005 to 2015. She also served as Scientific Director of a research institute on intellectual disabilities and autism spectrum disorder. Dr. Dionne has served as Principal Investigator on numerous research studies focused on early intervention and early childhood special education. In 2016, she began work as a United Nations Educational, Scientific and Cultural Organization (UNESCO) Chair on screening and assessment of young children, collaborating with Dr. Jane Squires and colleagues from other countries. Project objectives include training graduate students and conducting research activities in early intervention for children from birth to 6 years of age who are at risk for or have disabilities.

Jennifer Grisham, Ed.D., Professor, Interdisciplinary Early Childhood Education Program, and Director, Early Childhood Laboratory School, Department of Early Childhood, Special Education, and Counselor Education, College of Education, University of Kentucky, Lexington

Dr. Grisham is Professor in the Interdisciplinary Early Childhood Education program at the University of Kentucky, Lexington. She received her doctorate in education from the University of Kentucky. She is also Faculty Director of the Early Childhood Laboratory at the University of Kentucky, an inclusive early childhood program for children from birth to 5 years of age.

Dr. Grisham has directed research projects on topics including linking assessment and instruction, early care and education program quality, and individualizing instruction for young children with disabilities. In addition, she has conducted research on the effectiveness of instructional procedures that are embedded into developmentally appropriate activities, the application of multi-tiered systems of support in early childhood settings, and coaching teachers and caregivers to implement evidence-based instructional strategies with fidelity. Dr. Grisham is Project Director for the Kentucky Deaf-Blind Project, which provides technical assistance to families and service providers of infants, toddlers, children, and youth with deaf-blindness. She coauthored a book titled *Reach for the Stars: Planning for the Future* (with D. Haynes; American Printing House for the Blind, 2013), which is used to support families of young children in planning for their children's future and articulating their priorities to educational team members, as well as *Blended Practices for Teaching Young Children in Inclusive Settings, Second Edition* (with M. L. Hemmeter; Brookes Publishing Co., 2017), and *Assessing Young Children in Inclusive Settings: The Blended Practices Approach* (with K. Pretti-Frontczak; Brookes Publishing Co., 2011). Finally, Dr. Grisham directed the nationwide field test for AEPS-3. Dr. Grisham is frequently asked to provide professional development to state departments of education, universities, and local education agencies on topics for which she conducts research throughout the country. Dr. Grisham is co-founder of a children's home and preschool program in Guatemala City, Hope for Tomorrow, where she accompanies students for the education abroad program. Dr. Grisham also works internationally in other locations to promote inclusion of young children with disabilities.

JoAnn (JJ) Johnson, Ph.D., Professor and Department Chair, Department of Child and Family Studies, College of Education, St. Cloud State University, Minnesota

Dr. Johnson is Professor in Child and Family Studies at St. Cloud State University in Minnesota, where she provides professional development education in early childhood education, early intervention, and early childhood special education. She completed her undergraduate degree in special education and elementary education at the University of Idaho and her master's and doctoral degrees in early intervention at the University of Oregon under the advisement of Dr. Diane Bricker.

Dr. Johnson has worked at University Centers for Excellence in Developmental Disabilities in Louisiana, Oregon, and Nevada as Program Coordinator, Teacher, Service Coordinator, Grant and Contract Administrator, Director, Principal Investigator, and Instructor. She served as Director of the Research and Educational Planning Center and the Nevada University Center for Excellence in Developmental Disabilities from 2001 to 2008, where she developed and administered lifespan programs, services, and supports for individuals with disabilities and their families. Her professional experiences encompass all service settings for young children, including neonatal intensive care units, pediatric intensive care units, well-baby clinics, home- and center-based programs for infants and young children (including Head Start and Early Head Start), nursing homes, supported employment, transition programs, special education schools, and university lab school programs. Much of her professional career has focused on developing and refining assessment and curriculum systems to support interventions for young children with disabilities, birth to age 6, and their families. Dr. Johnson is author, developer, and trainer of *An Activity-Based Approach to Early Intervention, Fourth Edition* (with N. Rahn & D. Bricker; Brookes Publishing Co., 2015), and the *Assessment, Evaluation, and Programming System for Infants and Children* (*AEPS*; Brookes Publishing Co., 2002, 2022) and has been involved with the system since her days as a graduate student at the University of Oregon. In her spare time, Dr. Johnson likes to read, work on home projects, observe and interact with young children, and support human and animal rights.

Marisa Macy, Ph.D., Cille and Ron Williams Endowed Community Chair for Early Childhood Education and Associate Professor, Early Childhood Education, College of Education, University of Nebraska at Kearney

Dr. Macy teaches early childhood classes at the University of Nebraska at Kearney. She does research related to young children with disabilities. Dr. Macy engages in research and outreach with the Buffett Early Childhood Institute. As the Community Chair, Dr. Macy adopts an integrated approach to early childhood education and development through theory, research, and practice that links empirical research with the creation of programs, ideas, and tools for practitioners and community members. She received master's and doctoral degrees in special education from the University of Oregon with an emphasis on early intervention and early childhood special education. Her research interests include assessment of children from birth to age 8 with delays, developmental screening, play, and personnel preparation.

Kristine Slentz, Ph.D., Professor Emerita, Department of Special Education and Education Leadership, Woodring College of Education, Western Washington University, Bellingham

Dr. Slentz began her career in early intervention and early childhood special education with home visiting and classroom teaching with infants, toddlers, and preschoolers and progressed to directing a regional home-based early intervention program in Montana. For decades, she was involved in preservice preparation of early interventionists and early childhood special educators at the University of Oregon and Western Washington University. She also provided technical assistance and program development for Part C in Washington. She is currently Professor Emeritus in the Department of Special Education at Western Washington University.

Dr. Slentz's involvement with AEPS began with the earliest versions of the system and continues today, including development, consultation, research, and training. Her particular areas of interest and expertise are assessment and evaluation, infant development, early intervention, and working within family contexts across cultures. She has been fortunate to combine her love of travel with international training and consultation opportunities in Canada, United Arab Emirates, Singapore, and Kenya.

Misti Waddell, M.S., Senior Research Assistant and Supervisor, Early Intervention Program, College of Education, University of Oregon, Eugene

Misti Waddell is Senior Research Assistant/Project Coordinator at the Early Intervention Program at the University of Oregon. She used the *Assessment, Evaluation, and Programming System for Infants and Children (AEPS)* in classroom settings early in her career and, since the early 1990s, contributed to the development and research of the second edition of AEPS (2002), including project coordination for several field-initiated research and outreach training projects. Most recently, Ms. Waddell served as coordinator for the field testing of AEPS-3. Her professional activities in curriculum-based assessment also focus on the social-emotional development of young children. She coordinated the research study Project SEAM: Preventing Behavior Disorders and Improving Social Emotional Competence in Infants and Toddlers with Disabilities to examine the psychometric properties of the *Social-Emotional Assessment/Evaluation Measure, Research Edition (SEAM™)* (with J. Squires, D. Bricker, K. Funk, J. Clifford, & R. Hoselton; Brookes Publishing Co., 2014). She is currently part of the development team and serves as project coordinator for Project SELECT: Social-Emotional Learning in Early Childhood for Infants and Toddlers, a federally funded project to develop the curricular component of SEAM. Ms. Waddell provides training for early childhood teachers, interventionists, and parents in developmental and social-emotional screening, assessment, and intervention, including *AEPS, SEAM, Ages & Stages Questionnaires®, Third Edition (ASQ®-3),* and *Ages & Stages Questionnaires®: Social-Emotional, Second Edition (ASQ®:SE-2).*

About the Contributors

Ching-I Chen, Ph.D., Associate Professor, Special Education Department, School of Lifespan Development and Educational Sciences, Kent State University, Ohio

Dr. Chen is Associate Professor of Early Childhood Intervention at Kent State University. She is the lead translator of the traditional version of *Ages & Stages Questionnaires® in Chinese, Third Edition (ASQ®-3 Chinese)* (by J. Squires & D. Bricker; Brookes Publishing Co., 2019). She received her doctorate in early intervention/special education from the University of Oregon and was a university postdoctoral fellow at the University of Connecticut Health Center. Dr. Chen's work focuses on the development and application of culturally and linguistically relevant assessments and personnel development in early childhood intervention. She loves reading, traveling, and cats.

Naomi Rahn, Ph.D., Assistant Professor, Department of Special Education, University of Wisconsin–Whitewater

Dr. Rahn is Assistant Professor of Special Education at the University of Wisconsin–Whitewater. She completed her undergraduate degree in communicative disorders at the University of Wisconsin–Madison, her master's degree in early intervention at the University of Oregon, and her doctoral degree in special education at the University of Minnesota under the advisement of Dr. Scott McConnell. She has worked as a preschool special education teacher with children having a range of needs, including children with significant disabilities, and as an early interventionist providing services to infants and toddlers with special needs and their families. Dr. Rahn is author of *An Activity-Based Approach to Early Intervention, Fourth Edition* (with J. Johnson & D. Bricker; Brookes Publishing Co., 2015). While at the University of Oregon, she provided training on AEPS and earlier editions of *An Activity-Based Approach to Early Intervention* to programs around the country as part of an outreach training grant. Her areas of interest include naturalistic intervention strategies, early language and literacy interventions, multi-tiered systems of support, and personnel preparation. Dr. Rahn's research focuses on embedded vocabulary and language interventions for young children with disabilities and at risk for disabilities.

About EMRG

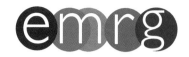

The Early Intervention Management and Research Group (EMRG) is a non-profit mutual benefit corporation that was created to manage future developments associated with linked measurement and curriculum systems designed to enhance early childhood intervention offered to young children and their families. EMRG has two general objectives: 1) oversee the future development of AEPS®, and 2) conduct descriptive and empirical research to refine and enhance AEPS.

For more information about EMRG and ongoing research, see https://aeps-emrg.weebly.com/.

EMRG BOARD MEMBERS

*To teachers, children, and families of the University
of Kentucky Early Childhood Laboratory who conceptualized,
assisted in writing, and validated the AEPS-3 Curriculum, thank
you for implementing high-quality inclusive programming for ALL young
children and serving as a model for the community, the state, and the nation*

I

AEPS®-3 Curriculum Organization and Use

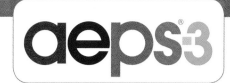

1

AEPS®-3 Curriculum Foundations and Framework

The AEPS-3 Curriculum is grounded in established contemporary early childhood developmental theory as well as recommended practices in early intervention and early childhood special education (EI/ECSE). The AEPS-3 Curriculum is a core component of AEPS-3 and a key part of the AEPS-3 *linked system.* It is specifically designed to be used as part of a multi-tiered system of support in all early childhood settings. Figure 1.1 illustrates the linked system approach that underlies AEPS-3.

As a complete system, AEPS-3 directly links the components of *assessment, goal/outcome development, teaching/intervention,* and *progress monitoring.* A linked system is one that allows practitioners to collect assessment data and use those data to develop specific developmental and academic goals, plan teaching/intervention efforts, and guide monitoring of children's progress.

AEPS-3 is such a system. Within it, the AEPS-3 Curriculum provides content for and guidance on what and how to teach individuals and groups of children (infants, toddlers, and preschoolers) who are learning at different levels and who acquire new skills and information in different ways. Throughout the AEPS-3 Curriculum, the term *children* is used to refer to the age range that includes infants, toddlers, and preschoolers. The *curriculum* content and procedures offer teachers, interventionists, and specialists detailed guidance about how to do the following:

- Collect initial assessment information to establish children's developmental skills and informational levels in all important areas.

- Use assessment data to make instructional/programming decisions about outcomes to teach within hierarchical sequences of developmental and content skills. Program development at this level provides a clear, appropriate scope and sequence of what to teach.

- Teach skills embedded within regularly occurring routines and activities at home and in classrooms or other environments, using a range of evidence-based practices. Specifically, intervention and instructional strategies show how to effectively teach

  - All children individually and in groups

  - Some children who need extra help

  - Few children who have specialized needs that require individual supports

- Monitor progress using the AEPS-3 Test to determine whether teaching/intervention efforts have resulted in positive outcomes for individuals and groups of children.

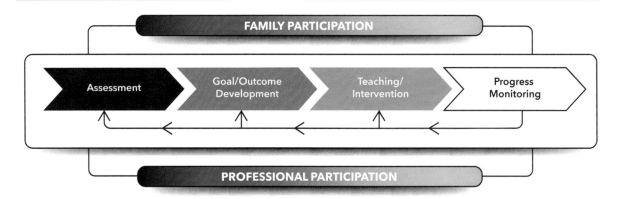

Figure 1.1. AEPS-3 Linked System Approach. This figure illustrates the conceptual framework of the AEPS-3 linked system. The arrow shapes represent the four main components of the AEPS-3 Linked System Framework: assessment, goal/outcome development, teaching/intervention, and progress monitoring. As the direction of the arrows illustrates, assessment informs goal/outcome development, goal/outcome development influences teaching/intervention, teaching/intervention informs progress monitoring, and progress monitoring then influences all three of the other parts. Participation of the family and professionals is essential throughout.

FOUNDATIONS

Designed for practitioners, the AEPS-3 Curriculum is based on three interrelated themes consistently found in recommended practices for infants and young children:

1. <u>MTSS</u>—The curriculum is organized as a *multi-tiered system of support (MTSS)* that provides specific strategies to meet the developmental needs of every child, regardless of the level of support necessary to promote effective learning.

2. <u>Blended practices</u>—The curriculum blends theory, strategies, and practices from early childhood education and early childhood special education (ECE/ECSE) to meet the needs of diverse groups of young children.

3. <u>ABI</u>—The curriculum uses *activity-based intervention (ABI)* as a strategy for providing teaching/intervention in the context of naturally occurring, *developmentally appropriate* routines and activities.

Each of these practices can support practitioners who serve infants and young children in home and classroom settings. The next section explains them in more detail.

1. Multi-tiered System of Support

The AEPS-3 Curriculum is designed to address the need for a continuum of differentiated strategies to effectively serve diverse groups of young children. Although MTSS has been around for some time as a means of offering different levels or intensities of teaching/intervention support, the notion of MTSS in early childhood emerged from discussions about how to apply response to intervention (RTI) in early childhood programs.

In 2019, the Division of Early Childhood (DEC) developed a position paper to address issues associated with MTSS in early childhood. As defined in the paper, MTSS "is a system-wide framework for delivering effective and efficient educational services and supports, matched to the needs of all learners for acquisition of essential skills, knowledge and dispositions, resulting in improved learner performance across one or more settings" (DEC, in press).

According to Carta and Miller Young (2019), the following principles characterize early childhood MTSS:

1. All children can learn and achieve when they are provided with high-quality services and supports to match their needs.

2. Instruction should focus on academic, social-emotional, and behavioral goals.

3. Children showing signs of delay should be identified as early as possible and provided with a level of instructional intensity to match their needs.

4. Interventions to address children's needs should be designed by collaborative teams that include parents, administrators, teachers, and other instructional staff. These interventions should be guided by student data and informed by evidence-based practices.

5. Children's responses to intervention should be monitored continuously, and explicit data-based decision rules should be in place for making adjustments in intervention.

6. All intervention should be based on evidence-based practice implemented with fidelity.

The AEPS-3 Curriculum is designed to meet the definition of an MTSS that helps teams differentiate approaches or levels of support for young children with diverse needs. Other widely known MTSS approaches include the Pyramid Model (Hemmeter et al., 2016), Recognition and Response (Coleman et al., 2006), and Building Blocks (Sandall et al., 2019).

2. Blended Practices

The term *blended practices* refers to "the integration of practices that can be used to address the needs of all children in inclusive settings" (Grisham-Brown & Hemmeter, 2017, p. 7). Practices that blend theories, strategies, and supports from general and special education are essential to effectively addressing the increasing diversity in contemporary early childhood settings. The AEPS-3 Curriculum draws from traditional child development theories such as Piaget's (1955) cognitive developmental theory and Bronfenbrenner's (1994) ecological systems theory, as well as behavioral principles such as Skinner's (1953) theory of behavior, that serve as the foundation for effective teaching/intervention practices in special education.

The AEPS-3 Curriculum draws on the work of Grisham-Brown and Hemmeter (2017), who proposed a curriculum framework based on identifying appropriate outcomes for all, some, and individual children. Goals/outcomes at each curriculum level are matched with detailed teaching/intervention strategies that provide increasing support:

- *Universal strategies* appropriate for teaching all children

- *Focused strategies* for targeted instructional outcomes

- *Specialized strategies* for children who require individualized support

The curriculum framework suggests a set of practices that serves as the foundation in any early childhood setting for helping children acquire common outcomes such as early learning standards—practices that rely on positive interactions between children and adults, a well-organized learning environment, and young children's hands-on learning.

3. Activity-Based Intervention

The AEPS-3 Curriculum includes an emphasis on delivering intervention/instruction that is derived largely from the four basic elements of ABI (Johnson et al., 2015):

1. ABI makes use of three types of activities:

   - Child-initiated activities, such as learning centers and free play

   - Regularly occurring routines, such as meals and transitions

   - Small-group activities that adults plan and guide, such as storytime

2. ABI encourages multiple and varied learning opportunities so that teaching occurs with sufficient frequency and across a variety of people and materials to support generalization of skills.

3. Functional and generative goals increase children's independence and allow them to use a variety of responses across settings.

4. ABI uses consequences that are natural or logical to the task to provide immediate and relevant feedback as children learn new skills.

Table 1.1. Evidence-based practices and skill areas

Evidence-based practice	Skill area(s) aligned with practice
Differential reinforcement	Play, engagement, and appropriate behavior
Correspondence training	Engagement, play, academic skills, and health/safety skills
High-probability requests	Request-following, social skills, and communication skills
Modeling, mand-modeling, incidental teaching, and naturalistic time delay (milieu teaching)	Requesting, choice making, saying/signing single/multiple words, play expansions, and responding to questions
Graduated guidance	Safety skills, feeding self, and dressing
System of least prompts	Play skills and dressing
Constant time delay Progressive time delay	Play skills, academic skills (counting, reading), prewriting, engagement, peer imitation, and communication skills
Simultaneous prompting	Play skills and home skills
Peer-mediated instruction	Social skills

Other Evidence-Based Practices (EBP)

The AEPS-3 Curriculum incorporates a variety of evidence-based teaching/intervention practices in ECE/ECSE, defined as "practices and programs shown by high-quality research to have meaningful effects on student outcomes" (Cook & Odom, 2013, p. 135). The AEPS-3 Curriculum uses principles and research-based strategies associated with such evidence-based practices as embedded instruction, *data-driven decision making (DDDM)*, and specific systematic instruction, each of which is addressed in the paragraphs that follow. Table 1.1 lists the strategies identified throughout the AEPS-3 Curriculum along with the skills that are best aligned with each strategy.

Embedded Instruction. Embedded instruction occurs when a child is engaged in preferred activities and an adult intentionally uses that activity as an opportunity to practice or demonstrate a target skill by expanding, modifying, or taking a logical next step with the skill. The activity itself provides feedback based on the child's response. Embedded instruction, which is an underlying process of ABI, has been shown repeatedly to be an effective method for helping infants and young children with and without disabilities acquire or expand skills. Embedded instruction has been used successfully to teach preacademic, social, communication, motor, adaptive, and cognitive skills to young children. The AEPS-3 Curriculum embeds all AEPS-3 Test items in commonly occurring routines and activities that take place at home or in center-based environments such as child care and pre-K classrooms.

Data-Driven Decision Making. Data on individual children's performance levels are the best source of information for selecting appropriate teaching/intervention goals and effective teaching strategies matched to support needs. AEPS-3 is structured to provide evidence to guide decision making at each step in the linked system. Observing young children as they engage in daily activities yields a vast amount of information about what a child knows and is able to do over time. The AEPS-3 Test provides precise performance data to inform decisions about the most appropriate goals and objectives for each child. Likewise, data collected during teaching/intervention reveal information that is critical for adjusting outcomes and modifying teaching strategies. Progress monitoring data also provide updates to the assessment data from the test, forming a comprehensive profile of skills acquired across all areas of development.

Specific Systematic Instruction. The teaching strategies in the AEPS-3 Curriculum were selected because evidence demonstrates that they result in positive outcomes for young children who have disabilities or are at risk. Emerging evidence also indicates that some strategies (such as peer-mediated instruction and system of least prompts) are effective in teaching high-priority skills to children without disabilities.

CURRICULUM FRAMEWORK

The AEPS-3 Curriculum is designed intentionally to coordinate and integrate recommended practices and evidence-based research into a coherent, easy-to-use framework by suggesting differentiated instruction similar to an MTSS model, using evidence-based practices from both ECE and ECSE, and embedding those practices into home and classroom routines and activities. The sections that follow provide details about the curriculum's central elements and characteristics.

Inclusive of All Children From Birth to 6 Years, With and Without Disabilities

The AEPS-3 Curriculum makes it possible to teach critical early skills to all children. It should be useful for individual children in Early Head Start, children in Part C Early Intervention home settings, and groups of young children in preschool classrooms (blended, inclusive, or self-contained), including those with developmental and early academic problems who have not yet been formally identified for special services.

Based in Routines and Activities

The AEPS-3 Curriculum focuses on teaching during regularly occurring routines and activities at home and in the classroom. The curriculum is organized into 18 routines and activities (see Box 1.1 for a complete list) and emphasizes play and young children's successful participation in homes and classrooms. Practitioners use evidence-based strategies to teach specific developmental skills without removing young children from their daily routines and ongoing interactions with peers and family members.

Active & Outdoor Play	Field Trips
Arrival & Departure	Math
Art	Meals & Snacks
Bath Time	Music & Movement
Blocks	Nap & Sleep
Circle Time	Science (in Growing and Ready levels)
Diapering, Toileting, & Handwashing	Sensory
Dramatic Play	Technology (in Growing and Ready levels)
Dressing	Writing

Box 1.1 AEPS-3 Curriculum Routines and Activities

Organized Around Three Skill Ranges—Beginning, Growing, and Ready

In the curriculum, AEPS-3 items are grouped into three levels, making it possible to teach infants and young children developmental skills that are embedded in a consistent set of daily routines and activities. In early development, the times at which specific skills emerge differ from child to child, and some skill areas may develop more quickly than others for any given child.

The AEPS-3 Curriculum includes one complete volume for each skill level. Taken together, the three curriculum volumes provide comprehensive strategies for teaching developmental skills in each of the eight AEPS-3 areas to children who function developmentally between the ages of birth and 6 years.

- The Beginning level (Volume 3) includes foundational skills that *typically developing* children acquire in the first year to 18 months of life.

- The Growing level (Volume 4) generally covers those skills that require children to combine and apply earlier skills. These skills typically appear during the toddler years, from 18 months to 3 years of age.

- The Ready level (Volume 5) has more complex developmental and early academic skills that are typical of preschool-age children and considered important for success in school.

Tiered for Differentiated Teaching

The AEPS-3 Curriculum is arranged in differing tiers of support to help match teaching strategies to children's support needs. A central feature of the curriculum, this tiered model accommodates the varying rates at which young children learn skills in different developmental areas. This three-tiered model provides increasingly intensive intervention/instruction to help ensure the level of support needed for each child to participate successfully at home, in classrooms, and in community settings.

Each of the curriculum's three tiers of support—universal, focused, and specialized—contains a variety of suggestions for specific teaching strategies that are appropriate for children with and without disabilities. Figure 1.2 shows the tiered model of the AEPS-3 Curriculum framework in more detail, indicating for whom that tier's strategies are intended, the types of strategies the tier includes, and the frequency of data collection. As the figure shows, data collection occurs least frequently in Tier 1, more frequently in Tier 2, and most frequently in Tier 3. Refer to Figure 1.2 in the discussion that follows. The teaching strategies in Tier 1 are for all young children in high-quality early childhood learning environments. The teaching strategies in Tier 2 are for some children who need extra help, and those in Tier 3 are for the few children who need individual help.

Tier 1: Universal Support   The support strategies in Tier 1 reflect best practices in caregiving and teaching. They are designed to provide safe, healthy learning environments and high-quality, developmentally appropriate curriculum for ALL young children. Within the universal support tier, developmental skills constitute core curriculum content for infants and young children. Daily routines and activities provide meaningful teaching and learning contexts for every young child with or without disabilities. Each of the curriculum's routines and activities lists suggestions for the following:

- Arranging daily routines and activities

- Facilitating appropriate, positive social interactions

- Selecting materials

Universal strategies may not work well for every child, and some children may need alternatives that require more input and structure to learn specific skills.

Tier 2: Focused Support   The strategies within Tier 2 build on the routines and activities of the universal tier and involve relatively minor modifications and adaptations for SOME children who need extra help to ensure more frequent and focused learning opportunities. The AEPS-3 Curriculum offers a range of specific strategies for the following:

- Identifying targeted outcomes

- Adapting and modifying routines, activities, and environments

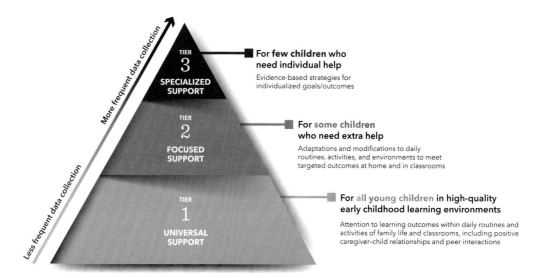

Figure 1.2.   Tiered Model of the AEPS-3 Curriculum Framework. This illustration depicts the three tiers of the AEPS-3 Curriculum (universal, focused, and specialized teaching strategies), indicates for whom the strategies are intended, and briefly describes the types of strategies included at that tier. Data are collected with increasing frequency the higher the tier.

- Incorporating child preferences, family priorities, and peer supports
- Selecting specialized materials
- Modifying teacher prompts

Tier 3: Specialized Support   Tier 3's specialized support strategies are for the FEW individual children who need intensive supports to address their unique learning goals, such as those found on IFSPs and IEPs. Specialized strategies build upon, rather than replace, universal and focused levels of teaching. Strategies at the specialized tier are individualized to help children acquire prerequisite and foundational skills more quickly and thus increase their participation in high-priority routines and activities. Specialized strategies emphasize the following:

- Suggestions for selecting high-priority skills to teach that emphasize positive *caregiver*–child relationships and promote peer interactions
- Specific individualized prompts and cues
- Materials and interactions that are specific to children with a variety of identified disabilities

Designed for Continuous Monitoring and Evidence-Based Decision Making

Monitoring children's progress is a central element of the AEPS-3 Curriculum, especially as they learn new skills. Monitoring children's progress is important for both teachers and parents and provides the necessary basis for making teaching decisions. Chapter 5 in this volume provides specific directions for matching how often to collect progress monitoring data with the level of teaching/intervention support provided (with data collected more often as the support level increases). The AEPS-3 Test's scoring system and organization are designed to allow you to monitor and track progress with precision as new skills emerge and children master them.

   Data that show children's progress (or lack thereof) are essential for determining the level of support children need to learn new skills. For efficiency's sake, it is important to move to new outcomes as soon as children master skills. Likewise, when progress monitoring data indicate progress is not occurring or is slower than desired, it is necessary to modify outcomes and/or teaching strategies. In the AEPS-3 linked system, assessment data are used to make decisions about selecting learning outcomes and goals for individual children, and progress monitoring data are used to move to new outcomes and goals and different teaching/intervention strategies.

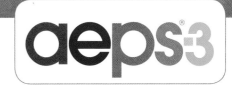

AEPS®-3 Curriculum Content and Organization

The AEPS-3 Curriculum covers eight developmental areas across the age range from birth to 6 years: Fine Motor, Gross Motor, Adaptive, Social-Emotional, Social-Communication, Cognitive, Literacy, and Math. The skills included in each *area* of development are the same for the AEPS-3 Test and Curriculum components. The curriculum embeds specific skills from each developmental area into routines and activities for teaching at home and in classrooms.

CURRICULUM LEVELS

For ease of use, the AEPS-3 Curriculum is organized in three separate volumes by developmental age or skill range: **Beginning, Growing,** and **Ready.** When selecting which curriculum level is appropriate, it is important to use AEPS-3 Test results to select the developmental content that is appropriate for each child.

Beginning Level (Volume 3)

Volume 3 contains the Beginning level curriculum. It includes developmental skills typically expected for infants and young children from birth to 18 months. The Beginning level contains the earliest skills in each of the eight areas, with a strong emphasis on early motor, social-communication, and interaction skills. Skills at the Beginning level are primarily foundational skills that are components of later, more complex skills. Following are some examples:

- Rolls from stomach to back

- Uses finger to touch or point

- Uses consistent approximations for words or signs

- Responds appropriately to soothing by adults

- Imitates familiar vocalizations

Volume 3 is a curriculum resource for practitioners working with infants and toddlers or older children who have significant disabilities. It is an ideal resource for professionals such as Early Head Start home educators and early intervention home visitors, who will find valuable strategies for teaching infants and toddlers with and without disabilities in the context of family routines and activities. As noted, the Beginning level also is recommended to meet the needs of early childhood special educators who serve chronologically older children who are eligible for services under Part B, Section 619, in blended, inclusive, and self-contained classrooms. The tiered, activity-based curriculum framework is effective for teaching a range of specific, developmentally early goals to very young children being served in a range of early childhood environments (such as child care). As a result, Volume 3 is a valuable resource for teachers and interventionists who are looking for help organizing routines, planning activities, arranging environments, selecting materials, and teaching specific skills in their infant classrooms and in infants' homes.

Growing Level (Volume 4)

Volume 4 contains the Growing level curriculum. It includes skills expected for typically developing older toddlers and young children, as well as older children with significant disabilities who are functioning at a developmental level from 18 months to 3 years. The Growing level includes the expanding, middle-range skills in each of the eight AEPS-3 areas and emphasizes social-emotional, early cognitive, adaptive, social-communication, and early literacy skills. Skills at the Growing level are basic, building on the earlier foundational and prerequisite skills targeted in Volume 3. Following are some examples:

- Jumps up and down in place

- Scribbles

- Uses 50 single words, signs, or symbols

- Meets behavioral expectations in familiar environments

- Indicates need to use toilet

- Identifies common concepts

Volume 4 is a curriculum resource for practitioners who work with older toddlers in home and classroom settings. Early Head Start home educators and Part C Early Intervention home visitors will find valuable strategies for teaching functional basic skills to young children with and without disabilities in the context of play and family routines and activities. The AEPS-3 Curriculum has been specifically designed to meet the needs of preschool special educators who serve diverse groups of developmentally younger eligible children under Part B, Section 619, in blended, inclusive, and self-contained classrooms. The tiered, activity-based curriculum framework is effective for teaching a range of specific, developmentally early goals and for improving the quality of routines and activities in any early childhood environment. Volume 4 is also a valuable resource for teachers and other providers who work with toddlers and who are looking for help organizing routines, planning activities, arranging environments, selecting materials, and teaching specific skills in their classrooms and in children's homes.

Ready Level (Volume 5)

Volume 5 contains the Ready level curriculum. It includes skills expected for typically developing preschoolers or children who are functioning in the 3- to 6-year developmental age range. Skills at the Ready level are the most difficult in each of the eight AEPS-3 areas and emphasize cognitive, social-communication, math, and literacy skills necessary for success in school. These skills tend to be complex combinations of basic skills contained in Volume 4. Following are some examples:

- Rides and steers tricycle

- Uses conversational rules

- Responds appropriately to warnings

- Counts forward to 10

- Names 12 frequently occurring letters

Volume 5 is a curriculum resource for preschool and kindergarten teachers who serve developmentally diverse groups of young children. AEPS-3 Curriculum strategies are especially useful for blended or inclusive classrooms that serve children with and without identified disabilities. The tiered, activity-based curriculum framework is effective for teaching a range of specific preschool goals and is designed to prepare children for kindergarten programs that follow developmentally appropriate practices. Because the curriculum strategies are equally appropriate for home and classroom use, the same skills can be addressed in the context of play, routines, and activities both at home and at school, promoting home–school coordination. Volume 5 is a valuable resource for classroom teachers who are looking for help organizing routines, planning activities, arranging environments, selecting materials, and teaching specific preschool skills in their classrooms and in children's homes.

CURRICULUM ROUTINES AND ACTIVITIES

The AEPS-3 Curriculum is organized into **18 routines and activities.** With the exception that the Beginning level does not include Science or Technology, the same routines and activities are included in the Beginning, Growing, and Ready levels:

- Active & Outdoor Play

- Arrival & Departure

- Art

- Bath Time

- Block Play

- Circle Time

- Diapering, Toileting, & Handwashing

- Dramatic Play

- Dressing

- Field Trips

- Math

- Meals & Snacks

- Music & Movement

- Nap & Sleep

- Science

- Sensory

- Technology

- Writing

For purposes of the AEPS-3 Curriculum, **routines** are common sequences of behavior that occur every day in homes and early childhood classrooms. Routines include Arrival & Departure; Bath Time; Diapering, Toileting, & Handwashing; Dressing; Meals & Snacks; and Nap & Sleep. **Activities** are more likely to be planned or facilitated by caregivers in specific locations and with specific materials and equipment. Activities include Active & Outdoor Play, Art, Block Play, Circle Time, Dramatic Play, Field Trips, Math, Music & Movement, Science, Sensory, Technology, and Writing.

Early childhood education can take place in many different settings, such as homes and classrooms, and AEPS-3 Curriculum strategies are appropriate for most settings. Some caregiving routines are equally relevant at home and at school, such as dressing, meals and snacks, and nap and sleep. Other routines are more common at home, such as bath time. Some occur most often in classrooms, such as science and math, although families can facilitate these activities at home. Others can occur at the playground or park, such as running and jumping (active and outdoor play). The AEPS-3 Curriculum emphasizes routines and activities that are meaningful and functional and focuses on teaching specific skills that promote participation and inclusion of all children.

Caregiving routines are highlighted in each curriculum volume and include Bath Time; Meals & Snacks; Dressing; Diapering, Toileting, & Handwashing; and Nap & Sleep. These routines are grounded in adult–child interactions during caregiving activities and are important to family life and sometimes to daily classroom schedules. Home educators and early interventionists often select caregiving routines that are high priority for parents as the context to address targeted skills. Specifically, in early intervention, caregiving routines serve as the foundation for developing *individualized family service plan (IFSP)* outcomes for young children with disabilities. In classrooms, caregiving routines often are closely related to program health and safety requirements and family-identified needs.

When children have difficulty participating in caregiving routines, the impact is generally high because of the importance of caregiver–child interactions, the high frequency of the routines, and the complexity of skills involved. Teachers in classrooms that have infants, toddlers, or older children with significant disabilities spend a considerable amount of time engaged in caregiving each day and need strategies for how to teach new skills in the context of routines. Children in preschool classrooms who can participate independently in eating, dressing, toileting, and naptime will have more time to devote to learning skills across other areas.

It is important to recognize the great variation among families in caregiving practices for eating, sleeping, dressing, and toileting routines, including but not limited to terminology and materials used and cultural traditions. Working on caregiving routines with parents at home means using as your teaching context the routines, terminology, and materials that are culturally appropriate for each family. Working in classrooms means knowing similarities to and differences between children's home routines and classroom expectations, as well as coordinating goals and strategies with parents.

Common routines and activities in early childhood classrooms tend to focus on prerequisite and early academic skills that are often addressed in learning centers and planned activities. Many of the AEPS-3 *Curriculum routines and activities* serve as the core of center-based classroom schedules, learning centers, and planned activities—for example, Arrival & Departure, Math, Science, Art, Writing, and Block Play. These are designed with emphasis on skills that promote success in school.

The 18 routines and activities in Volumes 3, 4, and 5 follow a consistent format:

- Name of the routine or activity

- Description of the routine or activity, including

  - How the routine or activity typically unfolds at home and school

  - Relevant developmental information across AEPS-3 areas

- Skill level/age range (Beginning, Growing, or Ready)

- List of *concurrent skills* by AEPS-3 area, with embedded learning opportunities as functional examples

- Narrative sections include the following:

  - **Universal Strategies**—Best practices for all children; Universal Strategies also includes two subsections, Interactions (useful teaching suggestions for all children) and Environment and Materials (overall suggestions for structuring the classroom environment and including materials that may be useful in teaching).

  - **Focused Strategies**—Strategies for teaching children who are struggling with a component of an outcome or whose development is stalled; these include a variety of relatively minor adaptations or modifications to help children catch up or keep up.

  - **Specialized Strategies**—Strategies for teaching children who need intensive support; these include a variety of specialized, individualized, and precise strategies.

Appendix A in this volume, Resources for AEPS-3 Curriculum Routines and Activities, provides additional resources to support the curriculum. The first section of this appendix presents lists of general resources to complement the curriculum, including books, journals, and web sites. The second part of the appendix is organized by the 18 routines and activities and includes lists of numerous complementary resources that are specific to each routine, such as articles and other readings, books, activities and ideas to try, and videos.

The AEPS-3 Skills Matrix in Appendix B spotlights individual skills by showing functional application across all routines and activities. Each skills matrix (there are eight total, one for each of the test's eight developmental areas) allows you to quickly and easily locate routines and activities that address specific AEPS-3 Test items. Ready-Set items are marked with a yellow flag.

In each skills matrix, the letter *B* corresponds with the Beginning level (Volume 3), *G* corresponds with the Growing level (Volume 4), and *R* corresponds with the Ready level (Volume 5). For example, the Fine Motor skills matrix indicates that AEPS-3 *goal* FM B1 (Activates object with finger) appears as a concurrent skill in 11 routines and activities. Most test items are linked to curriculum content in multiple routines and activities, which supports flexibility and opportunities for embedded learning. In this example, Active & Outdoor Play addresses the test item at both the Beginning and the Growing levels, as do several other routines and activities. Some items appear in more than one curriculum level because the emergence and growth of the skill occurs across a developmental span. As you plan teaching/ intervention efforts, consider which level and which routines and activities offer content best suited to children's needs.

Some test items on the skills matrix, such as the one in the example above, also have *Foundation Steps* (denoted by *FS*) that break a skill into discrete component skills. For children who have difficulty learning new skills at the level of individual AEPS-3 Test items, the Foundation Steps provide an even more granular breakdown of component subskills that are either a sequence of developmental precursors or steps in task analyses.

AEPS-3 CURRICULUM QUICK START

The AEPS-3 Curriculum is a go-to resource for dynamic, creative, differentiated early childhood education strategies. It helps practitioners

- Design routines and activities that use best practices at the <u>universal tier</u>.

- Plan and apply adaptations and modifications for children who need extra help learning at the <u>focused tier</u>.

- Implement specialized teaching for children who need intensive help to participate in ongoing routines and activities at the <u>specialized tier</u>.

The curriculum covers Fine Motor, Gross Motor, Adaptive, Social-Emotional, Social-Communication, Cognitive, Literacy, and Math areas across the age range from birth to 6 years. The skills included in each area are the same for both the AEPS-3 Test and Curriculum. The curriculum embeds specific skills from each of these developmental areas into routines and activities for teaching and intervening across multiple environments.

Following are the basic steps for choosing the appropriate curriculum level, identifying initial routines and activities, and identifying any supports that might be needed within each.

Step 1

Select the curriculum level that matches the developmental level of the children on your caseload or in your classroom, identifying whether you might need other levels for children who have more or less advanced learning needs:

- <u>Volume 3, Beginning</u>: Addresses early foundational skills (birth to 18 months developmentally)

- <u>Volume 4, Growing</u>: Addresses expanding skills (18 months to 3 years developmentally)

- <u>Volume 5, Ready</u>: Addresses complex, coordinated preschool and school readiness skills (3 to 6 years developmentally)

Step 2

Identify the routines and activities in the volume(s) that are **priority contexts in which children need to learn new skills.** Begin with those that

- Have been identified by parents and caregivers as difficult times in the daily schedule at home, in the classroom, or in other environments (such as a community outing).

- Contain skills from developmental areas that commonly interfere with children's learning (motor, cognitive, communication, social).

- Will help children with specific disabilities be more independent at home or in the classroom.

Step 3

- Identify any supports required for individual or groups of children within each routine or activity (the expectation is that at any given time, you may be implementing strategies from all three tiers). Keep in mind that universal strategies are appropriate for <u>all children</u>—children with and without disabilities, at home and in classrooms. The Universal Strategies section in each routine or activity chapter provides suggestions to help improve the flow of routines and the quality of planned activities. For example, this section addresses the best ways to set up diapering routines at home and in classrooms.

- Focused strategies are beneficial for <u>some children who need extra help with specific skills</u> at home or school, and for small groups of children in classrooms. The Focused Strategies section in each routine or activity provides suggestions that can help children catch up and increase successful participation. For example, this section suggests changes in materials, supplies, and interactions during art activities to address social-emotional, social-communication, cognitive, and literacy skills.

- Specialized strategies are individualized for <u>children who need intensive support</u> and focus on increasing access to and participation in home and classroom routines and activities. The Specialized Strategies section in each routine or activity chapter provides information about prompting, positioning, and adaptive equipment to address the needs of children who have specific disabilities. For example, this section suggests adaptive utensils to use during meals for children who have motor impairments.

In summary, AEPS-3 Curriculum aligns with AEPS-3 Test items across eight developmental areas at three developmental levels. It identifies concurrent AEPS-3 skills that can be addressed efficiently using 18 routines and activities that occur regularly within the lives of young children. The curriculum also provides detailed suggestions and examples for three tiers of teaching/intervention strategies within the context of the routines and activities. The remaining chapters guide providers in making decisions about what young children need to learn and how to teach and monitor progress toward acquiring and using targeted skills.

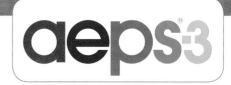

3

Deciding What to Teach

Selecting goals and outcomes—deciding what each child needs to learn—is the second component of the AEPS®-3 linked system. AEPS-3 gives you flexibility in identifying goals and outcomes for young learners. This chapter offers ideas for using the components of AEPS-3, such as the test and the *Family Assessment of Child Skills (FACS)*, to help you decide **what to teach.** Both the test and the FACS have their own instructions, which Volume 2 discusses in detail, so this chapter focuses on briefly describing how to use them to select teaching/intervention outcomes. As you read the suggestions offered, consider your particular program's assessment requirements. For example, some programs require providers to complete an entire *curriculum-based assessment* two or three times a year on all children, whereas others may require more frequent data collection but only in the areas of concern for individual children.

The AEPS-3 Curriculum's organization into routines and activities is designed to provide a range of flexible options for selecting goals or outcomes. The way the curriculum is used will vary depending on a program's philosophy, design, the population served, regulations, and the context in which services are provided. For example, if you are an early intervention home visitor or a Head Start home educator, for individual children, you will identify routines that occur regularly in the home and that are a priority for the family. In contrast, if you work in a blended/inclusive preschool classroom, you will select developmentally appropriate routines and activities that occur in your classroom setting, such as those for Circle Time & Storytime and Writing included in these volumes.

The AEPS-3 Curriculum is designed to allow professionals to address the learning needs of classroom groups of children, small groups of children, and individual children. In addition, the curriculum can be used as a standalone resource for any practitioner who is interested in implementing intentional strategies to teach developmental or content goals in the context of ongoing routines and activities, across a variety of settings.

DECIDING WHAT TO TEACH FOR ALL CHILDREN

Because AEPS-3 Test items align with many states' early learning standards and other program standards and outcomes, such as the Head Start Early Learning Outcomes Framework, implementing the AEPS-3 Curriculum allows programs to address important federal, state, and program goals and outcomes for specific groups of children such as children from birth to 3 years old who are receiving special education services or all 3- and 5-year-olds. To ensure that you are basing decisions about what to teach on sound assessment practices, AEPS-3 offers several strategies:

- **Use the concurrent skills for routines and activities:** One way to determine what to teach is to select outcomes from the list of concurrent AEPS-3 skills that appears near the beginning of each curriculum routines and activities chapter. Concurrent skills are AEPS-3 skills that can be easily embedded and taught during regular occurrences of each particular routine or activity. You can select what to teach from the concurrent skills lists, based on your program's standards and outcomes. For example, if you are required to address early literacy skills with all children in your program, you would identify the routines and activities that address specific AEPS-3 literacy skills (such as Art, Circle Time & Storytime, and Arrival & Departure) and focus on teaching those outcomes whenever the appropriate routines and activities occur during the day.

- **Use the AEPS-3 Test goals data:** Some programs require providers to collect assessment information on all children in their program. Completing the AEPS-3 Test can be challenging for providers who serve large numbers of children. Although some programs require providers to complete the entire AEPS-3 Test on all children, it may be appropriate to collect data at the goal level only, rather than including all the associated objectives. AEPS-3 Test goals can prove useful in making decisions about what to teach children who are typically developing when you have no concerns about their development—for example, typically developing children in blended/inclusive classrooms or infants and toddlers in Early Head Start.

- **Use the AEPS-3 Ready-Set:** The *Ready-Set* assessment contains developmental and content-specific skills that children need for success in early primary programs. You can use it to efficiently assess all children in their final year of preschool or first year of kindergarten. Select learning outcomes for groups of 4- to 6-year-olds from the Ready-Set skills the majority of children need to master.

- **Use the AEPS-3 Family Report and FACS:** The routines and activities reflected in the *Family Report* and FACS include the same skills around which the curriculum is organized. A routines and activities–based approach can help you select learning goals for any child at home or in a classroom group. As part of the outcome development process, you can engage families in conversations about the routines and activities that are priorities and concerns for them at home and in the community. First, locate the corresponding priority routine or activity in the curriculum, and then identify the specific skills children need to participate successfully in each routine or activity of interest.

DECIDING WHAT TO TEACH
FOR CHILDREN WHO DO NOT MAKE EXPECTED PROGRESS

As you implement the AEPS-3 Curriculum, you may notice that some children are unable to participate fully in the routines and activities or that their mastery of one or more associated skills appears to have stalled. To identify teaching outcomes to address these children's needs, you will first need to collect additional assessment information. Following are suggestions for pinpointing focused intervention/instruction to help some children learn specific skills:

- **Use the AEPS-3 Test:** If you have assessed only the AEPS-3 goals, conduct a more in-depth assessment by testing the objectives associated with the goals on which the child's development is not progressing. The child may need to learn a specific component skill before learning the more difficult goal. Conducting a fine-tuned assessment will help identify the specific skill components a child might be missing.

- **Use the Scoring Notes:** Go back to the developmental area(s) of the AEPS-3 Test where the child is not making expected progress and carefully review or collect precise data using the Scoring Notes. Some recurring issues associated with the skills might be causing the child trouble. For example, the child might be able to perform a skill only with particular people and materials or only in certain places. Or, the child might need a high level of assistance to perform skills correctly. Another possibility is that the child performs a skill, but the quality of performance is unacceptable. In each of these scenarios, you would need to focus your teaching/intervention on the aspect of the skill that is causing the problem (generalization, more independence, improved quality) rather than teaching a new or different skill.

- **Use the AEPS-3 FACS:** You can help caregivers complete the FACS in the areas(s) where the child is struggling to function and participate and then use information from the FACS to identify skills the family considers critical for successful participation in home and community routines and activities. Intervention/instruction can then focus on the specific skills both the professional and the family identify to give the child additional practice and support.

- **Group children with similar goals and outcomes:** You can use the assessment information from the AEPS-3 Test to identify small groups of children who may need to learn the same skill(s). By analyzing test data across groups of children, you are likely to see patterns that can help you design intentional small-group activities to focus on the skill(s) that several children need to learn.

DECIDING WHAT TO TEACH
FOR INDIVIDUAL CHILDREN WHO NEED SPECIALIZED SUPPORT

Some children may face significant challenges, such as the following, in acquiring the developmental goals and outcomes that all children need to learn:

1. Gaps in important milestones that same-age peers learned at an earlier age

2. Missing prerequisite skills that are components of more advanced skills

3. Issues that must be addressed before the child can move forward with learning new skills (specific disabilities or health issues, language differences, behavior challenges, food insecurity)

Children who are eligible for special services will have IFSPs or IEPs that list individualized goals or outcomes. It is essential that the team assigned to the child and family work together to develop a coordinated plan of intervention that addresses the child's disability, as discussed in Volume 1, Chapters 4 and 6. However, children not identified for special education services also may be missing prerequisites or developmental milestones, or they may have significant barriers to learning that must be addressed. The following sequence of steps will help you identify appropriate priorities for individual children. *Please note that these are steps in a sequence—NOT separate intervention options for determining learning outcomes.*

1. **Complete the AEPS-3 Family Report and FACS:** *Interview* the family to determine the routines and activities that are of highest priority in their family life. If the family has also completed the FACS, facilitate a discussion with caregivers to identify the specific skills the child needs to participate in difficult routines, and consider these skills when determining individual learning goals.

2. **Complete the entire AEPS-3 Test:** Assess all goals and objectives in the appropriate skill range across all eight areas of development, using the 3-point scoring system. The complete assessment will identify skills the child has **mastered** (those with a score of 2), skills that are **emerging** (score of 1), and skills **not yet in the child's repertoire** (score of 0). Analyze the results of the child's assessment data to identify any skills scored 1 or 0 over a period of time, and consider them as potential individual learning goals.

Occasionally, you may have difficulty identifying individual goals that are developmentally appropriate for children who learn new skills slowly or those who require specialized modifications and adaptations. For example, it might be difficult to identify specific AEPS skills to teach children with multiple disabilities (physical disabilities, sensory impairments). In those circumstances, **use the AEPS-3 Foundation Steps** to identify the incremental skills and behaviors that fall between AEPS-3 goals and objectives, and target those skills as individualized outcomes. These can be found in Volume 2, Chapter 3, as well as in the skills matrix in Appendix B.

3. **Cross-reference the AEPS-3 Test with data from the Family Report and FACS:** The Family Report identifies routines and activities that are priorities for the family, and the FACS identifies skills the child needs to participate in them. Compare the results of your AEPS-3 data analysis from step 2 with the results of the Family Report and FACS to identify two or three high-priority, maximum-impact goals and outcomes that meet all of the following criteria:

   - The goal is a priority for the family.

   - The goal will allow the child greater independence in daily routines and activities.

   - The child has not mastered the goal according to the AEPS-3 *criterion* (the child scored a 1 or 0 on the goal).

If both the professional and the family identify a skill as a priority, the child is likely to have many opportunities both at home and at school to learn and practice it.

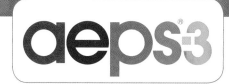

4

Deciding How to Teach

Teaching/intervention is the third component of the AEPS-3 linked system. Practitioners who work in early childhood settings make a multitude of large and small teaching decisions each day, because individual infants and young children learn differently from one another. The AEPS-3 Curriculum provides practical, specific resources that match a full range of teaching/intervention strategies with infants' and young children's individual needs. The AEPS-3 Curriculum is designed to include children with and without delays and disabilities and is designed for practitioners working in both home and classroom settings.

TIERED TEACHING/INTERVENTION STRATEGIES

The curriculum organizes AEPS-3 skills in 18 routines and activities, with each routine or activity further organized in three teaching/intervention tiers, as introduced in Chapter 1 (see Figure 1.2), that match specific teaching/intervention strategies to individual children's needs:

- Tier 1, Universal Support: Strategies at this tier generally entail best practices in early childhood education (ECE) for ALL children.

- Tier 2, Focused Support: This tier's strategies offer suggestions for relatively minor modifications and adaptations, often temporary, to help SOME children whose progress is falling behind their peers at Tier 1.

- Tier 3, Specialized Support: Strategies at this tier offer more intensive and individualized teaching techniques that are necessary for the relatively FEW children who are learning prerequisite or foundational skills or who are not progressing adequately with support of Tier 2 strategies.

Overall, teaching/intervention strategies become more intensive and intentional at each tier, beginning with a strong foundation of teaching for all children and progressing to more specialized and individualized interventions for children who need higher levels of support.

Several assumptions underlie this tiered arrangement:

- All children require a high-quality early childhood program with environments, materials, schedules, and interactions that facilitate learning (Tier 1).

- The teaching/intervention strategies suggested for Tiers 2 and 3 are cumulative—they do not replace the strategies at earlier levels. Tier 2's focused support strategies build on the foundation of Tier 1's universal support strategies, and Tier 3's specialized support strategies build on the strategies in Tiers 1 and 2.

- Children's problems acquiring skills and behaviors are identified early and targeted for specific teaching interaction, regardless of the types or levels of need.

- As much as possible, children with disabilities should be taught using strategies similar to those used for their peers and should be included in routines and activities with their peers to the greatest extent possible.

- Monitoring progress toward learning goals and outcomes becomes more frequent and specific as interventions become more intensive (see Chapter 5 for details).

The AEPS-3 Curriculum

- Provides increasingly frequent opportunities to learn within routines and activities for children who need extra practice to acquire skills both at home and in classrooms.

- Arranges more specific teaching interactions within routines and activities to match needs for increased structure both at home and in classrooms.

- Emphasizes adult–child interactions at home and at school and peer interactions in classrooms.

- Organizes teaching strategies for large groups, small groups, and individual teaching interactions in classrooms.

UNIVERSAL STRATEGIES

Based on child development and learning theories, the National Association for the Education of Young Children (Copple & Bredekamp, 2009) and the Division for Early Childhood Recommended Practices (Division for Early Childhood, 2014) have developed recommended guidelines for educating young children:

1. Young children learn best in the context of engaging interactive routines and activities.

2. The design of early childhood activities is most effective when it addresses young children's preferences and interests.

3. A program's sensitivity to the cultural and linguistic backgrounds of young children and their families is foundational for educational success.

4. Curriculum content and strategies should accommodate young children who are developing typically, those who are at risk, and those who have identified disabilities.

Universal teaching involves designing environments, activities, and interactions that create opportunities to learn skills that are important for success in present and future environments. Universal strategies in Tier 1 emphasize broad goals and outcomes, such as state ECE standards, that all children need to learn. At the universal support level, the AEPS-3 Curriculum provides recommendations for designing learning environments, selecting materials and equipment, and supporting social interactions. The Tier 1 recommended strategies embed a core set of early childhood goals and objectives in play, daily routines, and activities.

Physical and Learning Environments

Young children need a **schedule** of routines and activities that incorporates their learning needs. An ideal classroom schedule includes

- Opportunities for child-initiated and adult-guided activities

- Balance between movement and quiet activities

- Brief, focused activities

- Planned transition times when children are alerted to upcoming events

Consistent, predictable daily home schedules are beneficial and should include both ample opportunities for child-initiated activities and structure for learning during caregiving routines such as eating, bathing, and sleeping. Transition times at home also tend to go more smoothly when caregivers alert children to upcoming events that are outside of the typical daily routine. Children learn best when daily schedules are taught directly and implemented with consistency. In classrooms, a copy of the daily schedule should be posted, reviewed regularly, and referred to often. As at home, children should be alerted about transitions and unexpected schedule changes, such as those for an upcoming field trip.

Physical environments at home and in the classroom are best organized to allow children easy access to activities and materials while also maintaining health and safety standards. In classrooms, teachers generally create learning centers to cover all content areas, including art, blocks, dramatic play, math, music, sensory table, science, and writing. Learning centers should be designed around the interests of all children in the classroom, contain sufficient materials for multiple children to use the center at one time, and be arranged so noisy centers are separated from quiet ones. There should also be clear physical areas and visual boundaries for learning centers and limits on the number of children allowed to use a center at one time. Although families are unlikely to set up formal learning centers in their homes, young children still benefit from having access to learning experiences that include art activities, opportunities to engage with manipulatives, interactions with print material, and opportunities to express themselves through music, movement, and drama. In home and classroom environments, children need opportunities for active play activities both indoors and outdoors.

Materials

Developmentally appropriate materials give children opportunities to engage with their environments in ways that let them practice emerging skills and learn new skills. For young children, selecting and using learning materials can be a fun, dynamic endeavor that springs from everyday events and happenings. Following are some general suggestions:

- **Select materials that are based on children's immediate interests.** Children are more likely to interact with materials that reflect and expand on the most interesting aspects of their daily lives. For example, when children notice and talk about construction equipment near their homes or classrooms, adults can find books about construction and construction equipment, place toy construction trucks in play areas, or use simple art supplies (empty boxes, pipe cleaners, papers) to make construction sites.

- **Rotate learning materials regularly to provide novelty and increase engagement.** Children's interests change frequently, and when interest in a topic or materials fades, it is time for new supplies and activities.

- **Make sure enough materials are available for several children to play with preferred items at the same time.** When you realize a toy or material is a favorite, consider getting multiples of the item to prevent arguments, promote imitation, and encourage communication.

- **Choose objects that promote positive social interactions between and among children.** Young children can learn about turn-taking on a toy such as a rocking boat that safely holds only two at a time, whereas older children might take turns in a simple board game. Siblings can take turns helping set the table. Children will learn to cooperate if given opportunities to do so, such as by creating a shared art collage on a large piece of butcher paper.

- **Stock plenty of open-ended materials that allow children to use their creativity.** Young children do not need expensive toys to experiment, create, and manipulate. Scraps of material, empty containers, cardboard rolls, baskets, boxes, clothing that no longer fits, leaves, pinecones, shells, wallpaper scraps, and colored paper can offer endless opportunities for young children to engage in a variety of activities.

Social Interactions

One of the most prominent and pervasive aspects of universal teaching/instruction is the social interaction that occurs between children and adults and among peers. The ways adults interact with young children and support peer interactions create an important framework for young children's overall development. Positive interaction between young children and caregivers is one of the best predictors of later social competence with peers, and positive interactions with peers is a critical element of success in classrooms.

Positive Adult-Child Interactions   Trusting relationships with familiar adults encourage children to take chances in new learning situations and initiate their own learning opportunities. Strategies for developing nurturing relationships very early in life include

- Being responsive to infants' cues for attention, caregiving, and soothing
- Directing children's attention
- Naming and describing events, objects, and people in the environment
- Redirecting children rather than correcting them.
- Focusing on positive behaviors

Parallel strategies, once children develop language, are

- Following children's leads
- Having meaningful conversations
- Talking with each child at their own level
- Discussing topics that are of interest to each child
- Acknowledging children's efforts
- Giving children choices

To support a young child's learning, adults can engage in supportive practices that are known to encourage early learning, including teaching early concepts, providing feedback, and modeling language. Adults can promote concept development by asking children questions to encourage problem solving, creating opportunities for them to explore new ideas, and letting children try out their own solutions to common problems. Adults also hold the important role of providing ongoing, quality feedback, using whatever level of support each child needs to be successful and expand learning. Some of the most effective, convenient supports for learning at the universal tier are language modeling strategies that include conversations, open-ended questions, repetition and extension, self- and parallel talk, and introduction of new vocabulary.

Positive Child-to-Child Interactions   Teaching positive interactions between and among children is another important element of the universal tier. One way adults can support these interactions is to arrange for children who are less socially competent to engage in activities alongside children who are more socially competent. Adults can also create opportunities for conversation among children during routine activities such as meals and snacks. Playing simple games such as I Spy or asking open-ended conversation starters such as "Tell me about what you did this weekend" can create natural opportunities for children to converse with one another. In most situations, children will talk more to each other if adults act as participant observers, being in the immediate vicinity and keeping careful watch rather than being directive. When communication is not taking place, adults can briefly model what a child might say to another child ("Ask your friend if you can play") or provide a hint about what a child needs to say or do to interact appropriately with a peer or sibling ("What should you say to your sister when you want to play with a toy she has?").

To promote a positive early childhood social environment, it is essential for caregivers who interact with young children to have consistent social expectations. Experts agree that these expectations should be expressed as brief positive statements of what the caregiver wants children to do, limited in number, and focused on behaviors that promote and support a positive learning environment. Here are some examples of appropriate rules for young children at home or in classrooms: "Walk in the hallway." "Use your inside voice." "Be kind to each other." "Tell your friends 'good morning!'"

FOCUSED STRATEGIES

When a child's development is not progressing or the child is struggling to learn some component of a goal, you may need teaching/intervention strategies at the focused tier to provide more frequent, intentional learning opportunities. Focused strategies may also be necessary when families have concerns about a specific skill on which a child needs continuous practice or when a teacher becomes aware that a child is falling behind or is not performing a skill as expected. In the AEPS-3 Curriculum, the strategies identified as focused are temporary in nature rather than permanent modifications in teaching/intervention. This means that a provider might use them only until a child acquires a targeted outcome and then revert to more universal strategies. Some focused strategies can be used with small groups of children who experience learning challenges, thereby increasing the efficiency of instruction.

It is important to remember that focused teaching/intervention is delivered in addition to, and within the framework of, universal strategies, such as when a child fails to make progress and needs focused strategies in some areas but continues to learn much of what they need to know through the universal curriculum. The AEPS-3 Curriculum offers the following focused tier strategies to supplement high-quality universal strategies.

Using Embedding Schedules

When you need additional opportunities for teaching targeted skills, one of the best ways to ensure that children get additional learning opportunities is to create an **embedding schedule:** a matrix that depicts specific opportunities to practice the targeted outcome(s) throughout the day. An embedding schedule lists each targeted goal/outcome, along with information about how the outcome will be embedded into each routine or activity in a child's daily home and/or school schedule. Figure 4.1 presents a sample blank embedding schedule that can be used for individual children or small groups, in home and classroom settings. Take these steps when using the embedding schedule:

1. Identify the desired outcomes from assessment data.

2. Clearly define each desired goal/outcome and write a concise description of it in the space provided in the box at the top of each column on the sample blank schedule.

3. List all or a portion of the daily schedule in the boxes in the left column of the blank schedule.

4. Find where the child's or group's targeted goal/outcome intersects with an activity in the daily schedule. In the corresponding box on that row of the blank schedule, add a bullet that concisely describes the focused strategy adults will deliver to create an embedded learning opportunity.

Providers may develop embedding schedules for groups of children who are working on similar outcomes but perhaps different specific skills. A common example is when all children are working on identifying letters but each child is working on the letters in their own name.

Creating Easy, Effective Adaptations and Modifications

For children who need extra help, providing adaptations and modifications can increase attention, improve ability to follow directions, and promote independent participation. Following are some examples:

- If a child fails to pay attention during long activities, you might increase the child's chances for success by preparing shorter versions of the activities in advance.

- If a child has difficulty processing information when you provide task directions, consider giving the child additional time to respond after each direction.

- To simplify a task for a child or increase their independence in completing it, make available easier-to-use materials such as adapted scissors, chunky crayons, or puzzles with handles.

- Visual schedules can also provide children with information about what comes next in the day or the correct sequence of steps to complete tasks such as putting away materials or washing hands.

- Some children may be able to pay attention longer and participate more fully in activities when they have access to special equipment—for example, special seating such as a sensory seat, ball chair, rocker, or floor sitter.

- Other children might perform adaptive skills more independently if they can use adapted eating utensils such as bowls, spoons, or cups or if their clothing has elastic waistbands and Velcro fasteners to make dressing easier.

- Assistive technology can also increase children's independence—for example, the variety of available adapted switches allows young children to independently use battery-operated toys, small electronics, and computers.

Embedding Schedule

DIRECTIONS: This template can be used for individual children or small groups of children, in home and classroom settings. Follow these steps:

1. Identify targeted goals or outcomes from the assessment data.
2. Clearly define each desired goal/outcome, and write a concise description of each one in the blanks provided at the top of each column (one goal or outcome per column).
3. List all or a portion of the daily schedule in the boxes in the left column of the template.
4. Find the blank box in the template where the targeted goal/outcome from the top row intersects with an activity in the daily schedule column at left. In that box, write a bullet point that concisely describes the focused strategy adults will deliver to create an embedded learning opportunity.

Daily Schedule	Goal/Outcome: _____	Goal/Outcome: _____	Goal/Outcome: _____
	Focused Strategy	Focused Strategy	Focused Strategy

Assessment, Evaluation, and Programming System for Infants and Children, Third Edition (AEPS®-3), by Bricker, Dionne, Grisham, Johnson, Johnson, Macy, Slentz, & Waddell. © 2022 Brookes Publishing Co. All rights reserved.

Figure 4.1.   Sample blank embedding schedule. An embedding schedule is a matrix (table) that shows opportunities to practice targeted goals or outcomes throughout the day. It lists each targeted goal/outcome, along with information about how the outcome will be embedded in each routine or activity in a child's daily home or school schedule.

- For children who cannot communicate their wants and needs verbally, a wide array of augmentative and alternative communication (AAC) devices is available ranging from general use items such as iPads to specially designed Tobii Dynavox AAC devices. A variety of communication applications is available for the iPad, such as Proloquo2Go, iCommunicate, and Voice4u.

Forming Small Groups

Small groups are another effective focused strategy:

- For children whose learning has not progressed, a small group can be designed to provide efficient teaching opportunities in which each child receives a minimum of six learning opportunities in sessions lasting no longer than 10 minutes. Ideally, children in small groups should participate in random order, with no one child receiving more than two learning opportunities in a row in order to maintain children's attention.

- Small groups are also useful for children who are struggling to learn a similar skill—for example, several children who are learning the letter A.

- You may also use a small group to teach different skills to each child in a common activity—for example, when one child is learning to identify the letters in their name and another child is working on writing the letters in their name while engaged in an art activity.

- You can teach different skills to different children in the group—for example, during a literacy activity, one child may be working on letter identification while another is working on numbers.

Among the advantages of small-group teaching are that

- Children may also learn nontargeted skills from their peers in the group

- It is an efficient use of a teacher's instructional time

- Children may learn social behaviors that are useful in other early childhood play and learning environments, such as waiting for a turn, interacting with other children, and paying attention within the context of group activities

Using Peer-Mediated Instruction

With peer-mediated instruction, a competent peer shows a child how to perform a communication or social skill and reinforces the desired targeted outcomes. This strategy can provide assistance and motivation to children who are working on learning particular skills. Considerations for implementing peer-mediated instruction include ensuring that the peer has already learned the skill being taught, planning motivating activities that are of interest to the children, and training and supporting the peer. For example, if a child needs to be reminded to stay seated and remain on task during a large-group activity, a peer might be taught to tap the child on the shoulder and show a visual cue, such as a picture of a child sitting down, to remind the other child to stay in place during the activity. Another example is if a child needs to learn to take turns, a more socially competent peer could be taught to verbally and physically support the other child in taking turns.

Scaffolding

The focused strategy of **scaffolding** involves providing targeted assistance to children and then fading the support as the child no longer needs it. Scaffolding techniques include hinting, explaining, modeling, and questioning. For example, if a child's goal is to follow a social routine, the caregiver or teacher may give hints such as asking questions to help a child remember the next step ("What comes next?"). To ensure that scaffolding is effective, teachers must provide only the support necessary for the child to grasp a new concept or learn a new skill and then gradually withdraw that support when the child no longer needs it. To accomplish this, teachers need to make moment-to-moment decisions about how much support each child needs and when to withdraw it.

SPECIALIZED STRATEGIES

When children have needs that cannot be addressed with strategies from the universal or focused tiers, strategies from the specialized tier are needed. These strategies build upon, rather than replace, universal and focused strategies.

Specialized strategies are designed individually to address foundational and prerequisite skills or to address unique barriers to learning that prevent children from learning new skills. Many children with individualized family service plan (IFSP) outcomes and *individualized education program (IEP)* goals need specialized support strategies to make adequate progress. At times, young children without disabilities might also need specialized strategies to acquire a concept or learn a skill. For example, for children who have short attention spans, it is necessary to teach attention to task before teaching concepts such as color or shape identification that are taught to all young children in early learning settings. Similarly, children must learn pincer grasp and wrist rotation before they can feed themselves independently. Here are some helpful suggestions for selecting specialized strategies:

- Complete an AEPS-3 Test on the child. **Results from the assessment will help you identify appropriate individualized goals and skill sequences for teaching them.**

- Gain a thorough understanding of each child's specific disabilities and the implications of their effects on the child's development. Physical and sensory impairments alter how children receive, process, and respond to intervention. Providers should be aware of how specific diagnoses such as autism, Down syndrome, or cerebral palsy affect children's learning, as well as the specific interventions and strategies that have proved effective for children with those diagnoses.

- Get to know each child's learning preferences. This will help you choose individualized prompts, cues, and materials that will motivate the child to learn. Some other important elements to consider include

  - The ways in which the child prefers to receive new information and explore new materials (auditory, visual, tactile)

  - Appropriate wait times before expecting a response from the child

  - The most effective and appropriate modes of response (physical, verbal, technological)

  - Types of reinforcement that most effectively motivate the child's persistence, engagement, and skill mastery

ABC Design for Individualized Teaching/Intervention

Specialized teaching strategies require careful attention to three elements of each teaching interaction:

1. Antecedents (the conditions that set the occasion for a child to demonstrate the skill)

2. Well-defined behaviors and responses expected from the child

3. Consequences (the results of correct and incorrect responses)

Together, these three elements constitute **ABC design** (Antecedents, Behavior, Consequences) for individualized teaching/intervention.

Antecedents   **Antecedents** are the many varied circumstances that set the occasion for a child to demonstrate a desired skill or behavior. Providers need to determine ahead of time where to teach, when to teach, and what materials are best to use. Ideally, antecedents for teaching individual outcomes are integrated within existing environments and ongoing activities at home and in the classroom. In addition, the most effective individual teaching interactions include antecedents for establishing joint attention, delivering task directions, and determining how long to wait for the child to respond. Once the child is paying attention, keep task directions short, clear, and direct, with the general intent to decrease the length of time it takes a child to respond.

Specific Behaviors   Another factor to consider before using a specialized strategy is the **specific behaviors** that define correct and incorrect responses, including criteria for acceptable and unacceptable responses. For consistency's sake, it is essential for all the adults who use a specialized strategy to have a shared understanding about what constitutes an acceptable and an unacceptable response. For example, if a goal is to have a child initiate a social interaction, the provider needs to indicate which of the child's behaviors would be considered correct (extending a toy to a friend, saying, "Play with me"; verbally greeting a peer) and which would be considered incorrect (grabbing a toy from another child; hitting a child and saying, "Mine!"). Specialized strategies can be used to address all AEPS-3 Test items, because each goal and *objective* is written as an observable behavior with specific criteria and examples.

For children who have IEP/IFSP goals and outcomes that fall between goals and objectives in the AEPS-3 sequences, use the AEPS-3 Foundation Steps for functional and developmental task analyses that identify specific incremental skills and behaviors. These can be found in Volume 2, Chapter 3, as well as in the AEPS-3 Skills Matrix in Appendix B of this volume, where they are indicated by the marker *FS*.

Consequences and Feedback　　**Consequences** are what happens after the child responds. The child should receive immediate **feedback** for demonstrating the expected response, ideally because the environment is arranged so the child attains the goal via natural consequences. For example, if the child is supposed to say "more milk" and does so, receiving more milk is the natural consequence of demonstrating the expected response. If the child does not demonstrate the correct response, the teacher's role is to provide additional support to help the child demonstrate the expected behavior. For example, if the child doesn't say "more milk," the child's mother might verbally model the correct response and use a variety of prompts. These include but are not limited to

- Indirect verbal prompts (asking, "What should you do next?")

- Direct verbal prompts (saying, "Turn on the water")

- Gestures (pointing to the correct item)

- Visual or physical modeling (demonstrating how to write a letter)

- Pictorial prompts (showing pictures of the sequences of steps in a task)

- Partial or full physical prompts (putting a hand over or under the child's hand to perform a manual task)

Developing Intervention Plans

An **intervention plan** is a tool for designing specialized instruction. Specifically, the intervention plan

- Ensures that ABC sequences are embedded into ongoing home and classroom routines and activities

- Describes when, where, and with what the child will learn the priority skill and how to set the occasion for the learning (antecedent)

- Provides a clear definition of correct and incorrect responses (behaviors)

- Details what the environment, teacher, or peer is supposed to do if the child demonstrates a correct response (provide reinforcement) or an incorrect response (provide additional support or consequences). Figure 4.2 presents an example of a completed intervention plan, and Figure 4.3 provides a blank template to be filled in with the ABC sequence information needed to deliver specialized instruction. (See also AEPS-3 Forms USB for a blank template.)

Evidence Base for Specialized Strategies

A great deal of research has been conducted on teaching/intervention strategies at the specialized tier, demonstrating that the practices are effective and efficient for teaching children from birth to age 6 years, with and without disabilities. Generally, evidence-based strategies fall into three broad categories:

1. Consequence strategies

2. Enhanced milieu teaching

3. Response prompting procedures

Intervention Plan
aeps3

Date(s) completed: _3/3/22_ Person completing form: _Maria_

Program: _Bright Beginnings Preschool_

Child's name: _Alex_

Skill: _Initiate social interactions using tablet computer communication application_

Before (A = Antecedent)	Possible Behavior Responses (B = Behavior)	After (C = Consequence)
1. When: *Free choice* **2. Where:** *Student-chosen classroom activity center (blocks area, library, etc.)* **3. With what:** *Student-chosen materials (blocks, books, tablet with GoTalkNow app, etc.)* **4. How:** • **Establish joint attention:** *Join the child in play by taking turns with the activity (take turns stacking blocks in a tower and knocking it down, take turns turning pages in a book, etc.).* • **Establish a topic:** *Talk with the child about the activity using target verbs (teacher says, "Let's build," "Put the block on," "Push it down," "Read the book," "Turn the page," etc.).* • **Make a request in a format the child can understand:** *Interrupt the play routine and look expectantly at the student.* • **Wait for the child to process:** *Wait 5 seconds for the child to initiate using the iPad.*	**Correct response (+)** *Alex presses the correct button on the tablet to initiate the correct verb within 5 seconds.* **Incorrect responses (−)** · *Alex does nothing within 5 seconds.* · *Alex reaches for the toy but does not initiate with the button on the tablet.* · *Alex presses the button for an incorrect verb (selects READ while playing in the blocks area).*	**Correct response (+)** *Teacher continues play with the action Alex requested and provides verbal feedback specific to the request ("Okay, I will build a tower").* **Incorrect responses (−)** · *Teacher models the correct response (pushes the correct button) and says, "Do this."* · *Teacher waits 5 seconds for Alex to imitate.* · *If Alex does not imitate, teacher provides physical prompt.* · *Teacher continues playing and provides verbal feedback specific to the task ("You want to build").*

Figure 4.2. Sample completed intervention plan. An intervention plan is a tool for designing specialized instruction. It ensures that ABC (Antecedent, Behavior, Consequence) sequences are embedded in ongoing routines and activities; describes when, where, and with what the child will learn the priority skill and how to set the occasion for the learning (Antecedent); clearly defines correct and incorrect responses (Behavior); and specifies what the environment, teacher, or peer should do when the child responds correctly and incorrectly (Consequence). The sample plan shown here for a child named Alex focuses on initiating social interactions using an app on a tablet computer.

Intervention Plan

aeps3

Date(s) completed: _____   Person completing form: _____

Program: _____

Child's name: _____

Skill: _____

Before (A = Antecedent)	Possible Behavior Responses (B = Behavior)	After (C = Consequence)
1. When: 2. Where: 3. With what: 4. How: • Establish joint attention: • Establish a topic:	Correct response (+)	Correct response (+)
• Make a request in a format the child can understand: • Wait for the child to process:	Incorrect responses (−)	Incorrect responses (−)

Figure 4.3.   Sample blank intervention plan. This template is designed to be filled in with the ABC (Antecedent, Behavior, Consequence) sequence information needed to deliver specialized instruction.

It is beyond the scope of this curriculum to describe every one of the specialized instructional strategies associated with each of these categories. Collins (2022) and Grisham-Brown and Hemmeter (2017) offer detailed descriptions, and Table 4.1 provides an overview of specific teaching/intervention strategies for the specialized tier.

Specialized strategies also are available for working with children who have specific disabilities. Table 4.2 presents a partial list of disability-specific strategies. The curriculum also suggests specialized, assistive, and adaptive equipment and materials associated with each specific routine or activity.

Table 4.1. Teaching/intervention strategies for specialized tier

Category	Strategy	Use of strategy	Process
Consequence strategies	Differential reinforcement	Used alone or in combination to increase positive behaviors and decrease negative or undesired behaviors	• Reinforce the desired behavior and ignore undesired behaviors. • Reinforce an incompatible behavior–any positive behavior the child cannot physically do at the same time as the undesired behavior. • Reinforce a positive alternative behavior–any behavior other than the undesired behavior. • Reinforce the omission of the behavior, providing reinforcement when the child is not engaging in the undesired behavior for a specified period of time. • Reinforce a lower rate of the undesired behavior, providing reinforcement whenever the child engages in the negative behavior fewer times than previously.
	Correspondence training	Used to reinforce a child for verbalizing and carrying out a plan of engagement	• Prompt the child initially to verbalize how they will engage in an activity. • Reinforce the child for verbalizing their plan, and then reinforce again for actually engaging in the activity as verbalized.
	High-probability requests	Used to increase rate of appropriate responding	• Make three to five high-probability requests (requests the child is likely to follow). • Make one lower-probability request (a request the child is less likely to follow). • Make all requests in rapid succession.
Enhanced milieu teaching/ naturalistic language intervention	Responsive interaction	Used in combination to support language production during interactions between peers/ teachers and children with language delays	• Follow a child's lead when they look, point, move toward, or comment. • Comment on what the child is doing. • Respond to and expand upon the child's attempts to communicate. • Provide language models that are somewhat more difficult than the child's current level.
	Environment arrangement techniques	Used to increase opportunities and motivation to communicate	• Limit access to an activity or material (place it out of reach or in a sealed container) until the child communicates. • Perform an unexpected event or create a spectacle. • Provide insufficient materials for a child to engage in an activity.
	Prompting strategies	Used in various combinations to promote new skills in communication or expand on current levels of communication	• Provide models for the specific words, gestures, or signs a child is learning (modeling). • Give the child a direction to say or tell, and then model the response (mand model). • Wait a specific period of time for the child to communicate before providing a model/mand model (time delay). • Be aware and take advantage of a child's interests, preferences, and engagement to motivate communication (incidental teaching).

Category	Strategy	Use of strategy	Process
Response prompting procedures	Graduated guidance	Used to support performance of motor tasks by providing dynamic levels of physical support	• Provide physical prompts as needed on a moment-by-moment basis. • Provide the minimum amount of prompting needed to support the child in performing a task. • Increase physical support as soon as the child begins to make mistakes. • Decrease physical support as soon as the child begins to perform the task independently.
	Most to least prompting	Used to teach new and unfamiliar fine and gross motor skills	• Begin by using the most intrusive prompt a child needs to perform a new skill. • Gradually reduce support by using less intrusive prompts as the child begins to perform the new skill with full support. • Remove prompts entirely when the child can perform the skill independently.
	System of least prompts	Used to teach new skills when the child performs some parts or steps of the task more independently than other parts or steps	• Allow time initially for the child to perform the task, or a step in the task, independently. • Provide the least amount of assistance possible for the child to perform the task or step successfully if the child does not perform it after a specific wait time. • Gradually increase the level of support for each task or step after each wait period. • Use a fully controlling prompt, if necessary, to ensure that the child performs the expected response.
	Time delay	Used to promote a child's ability to initiate and complete tasks	• Provide a task direction and immediately provide a prompt that ensures that the child completes the task (0 second delay). THEN • Provide a task direction and wait a period of time before prompting the response by either: Waiting a consistent number of seconds before providing the controlling prompt (constant time delay). OR Gradually increasing the amount of time between the task direction and a prompt (progressive time delay).
	Simultaneous prompting	Used to ensure correct responses by interspersing training trials for skills with probes	• Provide a task direction and immediately provide a controlling prompt that ensures that the child performs the expected response. • Prompt the child to complete the task during all training trials • Conduct probe trials in which no prompting is provided (before and/or after training trials) to see how well the child can perform the skill independently.

Table 4.2. Specialized strategies for working with specific disabilities

Disability	Specialized strategies
Physical disabilities	• Positioning equipment (floor sitters, standers, side-lying support devices) • Proper positioning techniques • Adapted eating utensils and writing utensils • Nonslip mats to secure materials on surfaces • Sign language • Oral-motor techniques (consult occupational therapist or speech-language pathologist) • Accessible environments • Augmentative and alternative communication (AAC) devices • Assistive technology
Visual impairments	• Materials with olfactory or tactile features • Accessible environments • Tactile symbols and books • Objects with contrasting colors • Slant boards • Assistive technology • Hand-under-hand prompting • Extra time to process information
Hearing impairments	• Sign language • Frequency modulation (FM) system • Preferential seating • Picture schedule to assist with transitions
Deafness-blindness	• Calendar system to assist with transitions • Object and tactile cues • Tactile books • AAC devices • Assistive technology • Tactile signing • Haptics • Extra time to process information
Autism	• Picture schedule to assist with transitions • Social Stories • Noise-reducing headphones • AAC devices • First-then boards
Intellectual disabilities	• Extra time to process information • Picture schedule to assist with transitions • Social Stories • AAC devices • Assistive technology • First-then boards

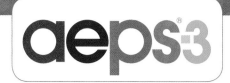

5

Progress Monitoring

Progress monitoring is the fourth component of the AEPS-3 linked system and refers to the ongoing evaluation of teaching/intervention effectiveness with individuals and groups of children. Progress monitoring data are used to inform future decisions about all facets of teaching/intervention.

Following teaching/intervention, teams need to determine its impact by collecting information to monitor progress. The AEPS-3 Curriculum is a tiered model of teaching/intervention with a tiered progress monitoring approach that requires more frequent and intense data collection as teaching strategies move from universal to focused to specialized support tiers. See Figure 5.1 for an overview of AEPS-3 progress monitoring. The sections that follow discuss the collection of progress monitoring data at each teaching/intervention tier.

UNIVERSAL (TIER 1) PROGRESS MONITORING

AEPS-3 offers several options for collecting progress monitoring data at the universal tier.

- States and programs typically align test items with state or agency outcomes and standards. Therefore, to monitor progress against state or agency outcomes, one option is to readminister all areas of the AEPS-3 Test two or three times a year. Because test content is aligned with state early childhood outcomes, progress on AEPS-3 Test items that were initially scored 0 or 1 and later scored 2 indicates progress toward state and agency outcomes.

- If your program does not require you to collect data on all state/agency outcomes or standards, and/or you are using AEPS-3 for children who are developing typically, you may readminister the AEPS-3 goals only or the Ready-Set two or three times a year.

- If you are a home visitor monitoring progress of children in homes, you may wish to readminister the AEPS-3 Family Report or Family Assessment of Child Skills (FACS) two or three times a year to get a sense of how parents perceive their children's progress toward participating in family routines and activities.

Data collected at the universal tier can be used to show children's growth over time as well as to determine which children need more intensive teaching/intervention and which skills or outcomes need the most attention. Teachers can use data collected at this tier to move children from universal to focused strategies on skills where an individual child or group of children is not making expected progress toward a targeted skill or concept. In summary, when using universal teaching/intervention, teachers or interventionists may readminister the entire AEPS-3 Test or Ready-Set, or use the Family Report or FACS to gather information about progress toward outcomes.

35

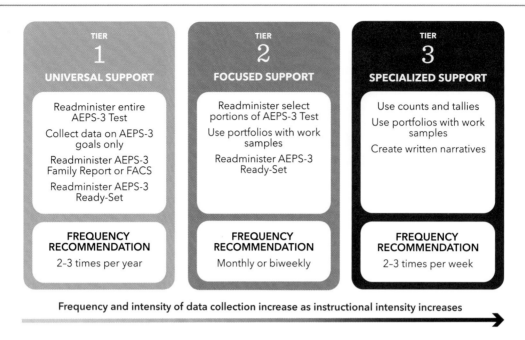

Figure 5.1.　Overview of AEPS-3 Progress Monitoring. This graphic summarizes the general guidelines and frequency recommendations for progress monitoring at all three tiers of the AEPS-3 Curriculum (Tier 1–Universal, Tier 2–Focused, Tier 3–Specialized).

FOCUSED (TIER 2) PROGRESS MONITORING

When teachers or interventionists use focused strategies, they are providing more intensive intervention than that in Tier 1 to support a child or small group of children whose development is not meeting expectations or who are not acquiring targeted outcomes at the expected rate. Using a focused strategy requires data to be collected more frequently and intensively than for universal strategies. The AEPS-3 Test is organized to facilitate data collection on specific skills at various levels of specificity and intensity. Following are some possibilities for monitoring progress when using Tier 2 strategies:

- When monitoring performance on targeted test goals or *strands* of skills over time, conduct a probe at least bimonthly or monthly. Figure 5.2 shows a sample AEPS-3 Test goal for alphabet knowledge that could be used as a probe for continuous monitoring.

- Another way of monitoring progress on targeted outcomes is to use permanent products (described in more detail on page 37) assembled in a **child portfolio.** Child portfolios can be an excellent way to document change and show qualitative aspects of developmental change—for example, the quality of a child's movement, or the time lapse between an adult's direction and the child's performance of the expected behavior. A provider addressing the alphabet knowledge goal shown in Figure 5.2 might collect work samples of the letters a child can write. A home visitor working with an infant might collect photos or videos of the infant using a targeted motor skill. It is important that any work samples in the portfolio include an anecdotal note stating the date of data collection and a description of the targeted skill.

- A teacher who is tracking the progress of a child's early school readiness skills could readminister Ready-Set. Done on a regular basis, this can provide information about targeted outcomes that continue to require focused strategies. As the child acquires the skills in Ready-Set, the teacher then incorporates those skills into teaching at the universal tier and collects data less frequently.

Data collected at the focused tier can also be used to make decisions about what level of ongoing support a child needs:

- If the child is making expected progress on a skill and further progress is still needed, the teacher can continue the focused strategy.

- If the child has mastered the targeted outcome, the teacher can discontinue the focused strategy.

- If the child is not making expected progress, the teacher can try other focused support strategies or consider designing more intensive strategies at the specialized tier to help the child learn the skill.

Strand C Alphabet Knowledge

 RS 29 ▸ | GOAL 1 | **Names all uppercase and lowercase letters of alphabet** Ⓡ

CRITERION: Child correctly states or signs letter name of all handwritten or printed uppercase <u>and</u> lowercase letters in English or other alphabet, presented separately in random sequence.

Example: When presented with random upper- and lowercase letters, child correctly names each letter in alphabet in upper- and lowercase.

Note: Items in this strand may be modified for other languages. Criteria can be adjusted up or down depending on the number of letters in the alphabet of child's language.

Figure 5.2. Sample AEPS-3 Literacy Area Goal for Progress Monitoring. The sample goal shown here could be used as a probe for continuous monitoring.

In summary, when implementing focused teaching/intervention, professionals may collect data more often by using AEPS-3 Test strands, Ready-Set, and/or child portfolios.

SPECIALIZED (TIER 3) PROGRESS MONITORING

Strategies at the specialized tier are used to help children learn foundational, prerequisite skills needed to acquire learning goals for the general curriculum and participate in daily routines and activities. At this tier, data must be collected frequently to determine whether a particular specialized strategy is effective.

For each goal taught using specialized strategies, target collecting data a minimum of two or three times a week. Three broad techniques used to collect the data are permanent products, written descriptions, and counts and tallies.

Permanent Products

Permanent products include items such as photos, videotapes, and written documents. Such products can be catalogued to evaluate changes in a child over time. For example, photos of a child sitting in a chair might reveal changes in how the child sits when physical support is reduced, and videotapes collected over time might demonstrate changes in how a child interacts with peers.

Written Descriptions

A **running record** documents all behaviors the child performs over a short period of time. This data collection method often is used when providers are interested in a child's social development—for example, teachers may observe a child interacting with a peer or sibling and record social-emotional and play skills. Running records also are used frequently when documenting children's language development. Teachers or interventionists may write down everything a child says while interacting with others during play or a routine activity.

Professionals also may write **anecdotal notes** based on observing the child demonstrating a particular goal during a specific event or activity. Anecdotal notes should be accurate, include the context in which the behavior is observed, and focus on the specific behavior. Teachers might use sticky notes or adhesive labels or make notes on an electronic tablet.

Counts and Tallies

Four types of counts and tallies help in collecting progress data on the effectiveness of specialized strategies:

- **Checklists** record whether a child performed the skill (marked with a + symbol) or did not perform it (– symbol). Take care not to overuse this common strategy because checklists often lack the detail necessary for making informed decisions. Customized data collection sheets are available for many specialized strategies, including time delay, system of least prompts, and mand model. Specialized checklists collect data at a detailed level, such as the exact prompt a child needs to perform a skill or whether the child demonstrates the behavior before or after a prompt. Such detailed data can be useful when making adjustments to strategies at the specialized tier.

- **Event sampling** is used to determine how frequently a child performs a skill when given an appropriate opportunity—for example, it is an efficient way to tally how many times a child initiates a social interaction or how many steps a child takes. When there is a need for more specific information than a simple frequency count would yield, the scoring notes from the AEPS-3 Test can be valuable. These notes can be used in several ways:

  - To describe a child's performance when skill quality is problematic

  - To identify when a child needs help to complete the goal

  - To specify when a child's behavior interferes with performing the skill

  - To determine when a modification is necessary to address specific learning problems

- **Time sampling** is used to observe behaviors that occur with high frequency. To determine whether a child has engaged in a behavior or performed a skill, the teacher or interventionist may divide the *observation* period into small increments and collect data at the end of each interval. For example, if the goal is to have a child participate with other children during small-group time, the teacher could set a timer to observe the child's behavior every 30 to 60 seconds.

- **Rubrics** help measure a child's generalized use of skills taught using specialized strategies. For each skill, a rubric usually provides descriptors at three to five different levels of successful performance. Table 5.1 shows a sample progress monitoring rubric that measures four performance levels (novice, apprentice, proficient, distinguished) and five criteria (performance, setting, material, people, embedded learning opportunities performed correctly).

Table 5.1. Sample progress monitoring rubric for a child's outcome

	1 Novice	2 Apprentice	3 Proficient	4 Distinguished
Performance	Struggling to meet expectations (baseline)	Approaching expectation	Meeting expectation (criterion)	Exceeding expectation
Setting	Across 1 or no settings	Across 2 settings **OR**	Across 3 settings **AND**	Across 4 or more settings **AND**
Material	With 1 or no materials	With 2-3 materials **OR**	With 4 materials **AND**	With 5 or more materials **AND**
People	With 1 or no people	With 2 people **OR**	With 3 people **AND**	With 4 or more people **AND**
Embedded learning opportunities performed correctly	25% or less	50% or less	90% or less	100%

With specialized strategies, it is necessary to collect progress monitoring data frequently, intensely, and precisely to allow team members to detect whether the strategies are effective. Teachers and interventionists should be prepared to continue using specialized strategies that help children make progress and to move to more advanced skills once children attain the criteria on skills that require specialized strategies. Conversely, teachers should be prepared to modify and replace specialized strategies if children are not making adequate progress.

In summary, permanent products, written descriptions, and counts and tallies are useful for monitoring progress when specialized teaching/intervention is employed.

AEPS-3 progress monitoring data collection provides information at each level of tiered teaching/intervention that informs every other component of the AEPS-3 linked system. Ongoing data collection accomplishes several things:

1. Updates initial assessment results

2. Indicates when goals/outcomes have been mastered or need to be adjusted

3. Informs providers and parents about the relative success of specific teaching/intervention strategies

As teaching/intervention strategies become more intensive and frequent, data collection also is increased in frequency and detail to match the level of effort and specificity invested to support each child's progress.

II

AEPS®-3 Curriculum Beginning Routines and Activities

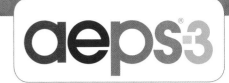

6

Active & Outdoor Play

Active & Outdoor Play includes children's participation in activities that help develop and use balance and mobility to acquire a vast array of motor skills (climb, ride, walk, run, jump, throw, kick, roll, swing, catch). The routines change significantly over time as young children become more aware of their environments (surfaces, toys, people, spaces) and interested in using materials in their active play, such as push and pull toys, riding toys, and playground equipment (balls, jump ropes, hoops and rings, climbing and hanging bars, slides and tunnels, swings, teeter-totters, merry-go-round, balance beam). The AEPS-3 Beginning level of Active & Outdoor Play uses skills from seven developmental areas.

Concurrent Skills

The following concurrent skills are AEPS-3 skills that can be easily embedded and taught during regular occurrences of Active & Outdoor Play.

FINE MOTOR Beginning Skills

A 1	Makes directed batting or swiping movements with each hand
A 1.1	Brings hands together near midline
A 1.2	Makes directed movements with arms
A 2	Grasps pea-size object
A 2.1	Grasps hand-size object
A 3	Stacks objects
A 3.1	Releases object into targeted space
A 3.2	Releases object into nondefined space
B 1	Activates object with finger
B 1.1	Uses finger to point or touch
B 1.2	Uses hand to activate object
B 1.3	Uses fingers to explore object
B 2.1	Turns object using either hand
B 3.4	Holds object with one hand and manipulates object or produces action with other hand
B 3.5	Transfers object from hand to hand

Embedded Learning Opportunities

- *Brings hands together while clapping during a song*
- *Picks up small pieces of cereal, raisins, or small crackers with finger and thumb*
- *Holds outdoor toys such as balls, shovels, animals, and chalk with hands*
- *Picks up toys and puts them in area designated by adult*
- *Uses fingers to point to objects in the environment, such as birds, trees, squirrels, and cars*
- *Uses fingers to explore things in the environment, such as grass, dirt, mulch, and leaves*
- *Holds bucket with one hand while using other hand to scoop sand into bucket*

GROSS MOTOR Beginning Skills

A 1 Turns head, moves arms, and kicks legs independently of each other

A 1.1 Kicks legs

A 1.2 Waves arms

A 1.3 Turns head side to side

A 2 Puts weight on one hand or arm while reaching with opposite hand

A 2.1 Remains propped on extended arms with head lifted

A 2.2 Remains propped on nonextended forearms with lifted head

A 4 Assumes balanced sitting position

A 4.1 Assumes hands-and-knees position from sitting

A 4.2 Regains balanced, upright sitting position after reaching across body

A 4.3 Regains balanced, upright sitting position after leaning left, right, and forward

A 4.4 Sits balanced without support

A 4.5 Sits balanced using hands for support

A 4.6 Holds head in midline when sitting supported

B 1 Creeps forward using alternating arm and leg movements

B 1.1 Rocks while in creeping position

B 1.2 Assumes creeping position

B 1.3 Crawls forward on stomach

B 1.4 Pivots on stomach

B 2 Stoops and regains balanced standing position

B 2.1 Rises from sitting to standing position

B 2.2 Stands unsupported

B 3.1 Walks without support

B 3.2 Walks with one-hand support

B 3.3 Walks with two-hand support

B 3.4 Cruises

B 6.3 Jumps down with support

C 1.6 Throws or rolls ball at target with two hands

C 3.3 Pushes riding toy with feet while steering

C 3.4 Sits on riding toy or in wagon while in motion

Embedded Learning Opportunities

■ *Turns head to track adult or object of interest, such as ball or animal*

■ *Sits to play with preferred toys*

■ *Pulls up to stand while holding on to age-appropriate climber or outdoor playhouse*

■ *Stoops and regains standing position while playing Peekaboo with adult through playhouse door*

■ *Walks supported by push toy on smooth surface*

■ *Explores outside environment while walking with adult with one- or two-hand support*

■ *Rides on riding toy with support from adult*

■ *Jumps from low landing on climber holding adult's hand*

■ *Throws or rolls playground ball with adult or peer*

ADAPTIVE Beginning Skills

A 4.1   Drinks from cup with spouted lid
A 4.2   Drinks from container held by adult
C 1.5   Takes off shoes
C 1.6   Takes off socks
C 1.7   Takes off hat

Embedded Learning Opportunities

■ *Drinks water from cup or water bottle with spouted lid with or without help from adult*

■ *Takes off socks, shoes, and hat upon entering classroom from outdoor play*

SOCIAL-EMOTIONAL Beginning Skills

A 1   Initiates positive social behavior toward familiar adult
A 1.1   Responds appropriately to familiar adult's affective tone
A 1.2   Responds to familiar adult's positive social behavior
A 2   Maintains social interaction with familiar adult
A 2.1   Initiates simple social interaction with familiar adult
A 2.2   Repeats part of interactive game or action in order to continue game or action
A 2.3   Responds to familiar game or action
B 2.2   Seeks comfort, closeness, or physical contact from familiar adult
B 2.3   Responds appropriately to soothing by adult
C 1.3   Plays near one or two peers
D 4.2   Claims and defends possessions

Embedded Learning Opportunities

■ *Smiles or vocalizes as adult approaches*

■ *Responds with excitement as adult uses elevated or excited voice to initiate interaction as they go down slide*

■ *Brings ball to adult in order to show interest in playing ball*

■ *Looks for and is comforted by adult when hurt*

■ *Plays with bucket and shovel near another child in sandbox*

■ *Indicates "mine" through gestures, signs, or words when another child takes their toys*

SOCIAL-COMMUNICATION Beginning Skills

A 1   Turns and looks toward person speaking
A 3.1   Vocalizes to another person expressing positive affective state
A 3.2   Vocalizes to another person expressing negative affective state
A 4   Uses intentional gestures, vocalizations, and objects to communicate
A 4.3   Expresses desire to continue activity
A 4.4   Expresses negation or protests
B 1   Follows gaze to establish joint attention
B 1.1   Follows pointing gestures with eyes
B 1.2   Looks toward object
B 2.1   Recognizes own and familiar names
B 2.2   Responds to single-word directive
C 1.3   Uses consistent approximations for words or signs
C 1.4   Uses consistent consonant–vowel combinations

Embedded Learning Opportunities

■ *Looks toward adult when name is called to gain attention*

■ *Uses speech sounds or word approximations to express enjoyment of an activity such as going down slide*

■ *Cries when something negative such as falling down takes place*

■ *Points at ball bin and looks expectantly at adult for help*

■ *Says "mo" to make request to be pushed more on swing*

COGNITIVE Beginning Skills

A 1   Orients to events or stimulation

A 1.1   Reacts to events or stimulation

A 2   Combines simple actions to examine people, animals, and objects

A 2.1   Uses sensory means to explore people, animals, and objects

B 1.1   Imitates novel simple motor action not already in repertoire

B 1.2   Imitates familiar simple motor action

B 2.1   Imitates novel vocalizations

B 2.2   Imitates familiar vocalizations

C 1.2   Locates hidden object

D 1.1   Uses part of object or support to obtain another object

D 1.2   Retains one object when second object is obtained

D 2   Coordinates actions with objects to achieve new outcomes

D 2.1   Tries different simple actions to achieve a goal

D 2.2   Uses simple actions on objects

E 1.2   Uses senses to explore

E 2.3   Makes observations

Embedded Learning Opportunities

■ *Looks to find source of sound such as dog barking or sirens from ambulance or fire truck*

■ *Walks or crawls to fence to watch lawnmower*

■ *Follows lead of adult or peer to shake parachute for first time*

■ *Uses toy shovel to dig in sandbox for toy animal buried by adult*

■ *Explores grass, mulch, leaves, or rocks by turning them over with both hands, looking from different perspectives, and smelling*

MATH Beginning Skills

A 1.2   Recites numbers 1–3

Embedded Learning Opportunities

■ *Says "1, 2, 3, go!" before sliding down slide*

UNIVERSAL STRATEGIES

These are best practices for ALL young children, with attention to meeting learning outcomes within daily routines and activities of family life and early childhood classrooms while promoting positive adult-child relationships and peer interactions.

Active and outdoor play in the very early developmental level involves infants and children becoming more mobile to readily access and explore their environment. Sitting, cruising, crawling, standing, and walking are all skills that allow children to explore. Adults are responsible for providing safe and appropriate outdoor and indoor environments for children to develop these skills. A safe and appropriate environment may include things like an age-appropriate climber, push toys, riding toys, balls, sand and water, and buckets and shovels. These materials should be in a secure place with surface materials and fall zones that meet safety standards.

Along with supporting active play and gross motor development, outdoor play provides opportunities for development of science concepts through exploration of different textures and materials, especially play with sand and water. Social-communication skills are easily incorporated into outdoor play by labeling items in the environment. Questioning and discussing novel things that are seen, heard, felt, and smelled outside supports developing conversation skills.

Interactions

Interactions with adults are a vital part of successful active and outdoor play routines for infants and young toddlers. Following are some suggested interactions for the Beginning level of this routine:

▲ Interact with children in a positive manner by using a pleasant tone of voice, smiling, and providing encouragement for new skills such as pushing a push toy or going down a slide.

▲ Incorporate opportunities to expand on children's vocabulary and early concepts by conversing with children and describing what is happening.

▲ Model both language and motor activities for infants and young children (throw or roll a ball, dig with shovels, open and close a door to a playhouse).

▲ Place children who are not mobile in a safe part of an outdoor play space, and give them multiple opportunities to experience the outdoor environment:

△ Place a protective cover on the ground atop both mulch and grass to offer children different experiences.

△ Give children a variety of items to play with (balls, plastic animals, buckets, shovels).

△ Walk children who are not mobile to different parts of the outdoor space to give them an opportunity to see more of what is around them.

△ Use peers, especially children who are older or have more skills, as a resource to teach young children. Children learn from peers by observing, imitating, and exploring the environment and play items together.

Environment and Materials

Following are some suggestions for environment and materials at the Beginning level of this routine:

▲ Ensure that the environment for active and outdoor play is safe—this is particularly important during infant and early toddler development:

△ Make sure outdoor spaces are secure and free from traffic.

△ Provide developmentally appropriate equipment, surface materials, and fall zones.

△ Use areas such as playgrounds and grassy spaces for active outdoor play.

▲ Vary the materials for active and outdoor play on the basis of location:

△ Let children explore sand and playground equipment through movement and sensory experiences.

△ Provide materials that are appropriate for active play in any safe environment (balls, cars and trucks, toy animals, riding toys, push toys).

■ FOCUSED STRATEGIES

These strategies are for teaching SOME children who are struggling with a component of a skill or whose development is stalled and who need extra help to catch up or keep up. The strategies include a variety of minor adaptations or modifications to daily routines, activities, and environments to meet targeted outcomes at home and in classrooms.

▲ Use repetition and consistency of environment and routine to help children become comfortable with and in control of the skills they are trying to master.

▲ Choose materials that interest children to help increase children's development toward individual goals by boosting their engagement and participation in an activity:

△ Select a favorite shirt to teach dressing.

△ Use favorite miniature toys to teach sorting and counting.

▲ Vary the environments where active and outdoor play occurs, using settings of interest to children to encourage them to practice their skills:

△ Practice sitting in chairs, swings, and on the ground for circle time.

△ Provide opportunities for running and throwing in the classroom play yard, at the park, and in the grass around the splash pool.

▲ Vary the materials used with children:

△ Give children time, if possible, to explore new items before they become involved in active and outdoor play.

△ Model how to use items, if necessary, to encourage children to become interested.

▲ Pay close attention for times when infants are comfortable, alert, and ready to learn or play. Some children may need time to warm up to new materials or games and may require many opportunities to watch and observe before becoming involved.

△ Learn to recognize children's cues and preferences.

△ Teach children who cannot speak to use simple signs (MORE, ALL DONE) so they can communicate their preferences.

△ Pair sign language with spoken words for children who are nonverbal or who have hearing impairments.

TIER 3

■ SPECIALIZED STRATEGIES

These strategies for teaching the FEW children who need intensive supports include a variety of specialized, individualized, precise evidence-based strategies to meet children's unique goals/outcomes:

▲ Give children multiple opportunities to express their choices for materials and activities in active and outdoor play.

▲ Let children choose items placed within their reach by using sign language or vocalizations and gestures.

▲ Use hand-over-hand support to help children with activities such as throwing and rolling a ball, digging in a sandbox with a shovel, or drawing with sidewalk chalk.

▲ Use verbal prompts to get a response during an activity (say "1, 2, 3, throw!" to let children know it is their turn to throw a ball).

▲ Adapt materials such as riding toys and push toys to make them more accessible for children with special needs:

△ Adapt the seat of a riding toy with a nonslip pad to help with stability.

△ Put something heavy, such as sand, in a push toy to make it more stable for supported walking.

▲ Include children with limited mobility in multiple activities during active and outdoor play:

△ Physically help a child go down a slide.

△ Place an adaptive chair inside an outdoor playhouse to allow a child who is not yet able to sit or stand independently to participate.

AEPS-3 Curriculum Resources (Appendix A)

Appendix A in this volume contains numerous additional resources to supplement the AEPS-3 Curriculum. The first part of the appendix presents a list of general curriculum resources, and the second part provides lists of supplementary resources for each individual routine and activity.

AEPS-3 Skills Matrix (Appendix B)

The AEPS-3 Skills Matrix in Appendix B of this volume spotlights individual skills by showing functional application across all routines and activities. Each skills matrix (there are eight total, one for each of the test's eight developmental areas) allows you to select individual AEPS-3 items for children who require an intensive focus on a few skills across routines and activities. For children who have difficulty learning new skills at the level of individual AEPS-3 items, the Foundation Steps (*FS*) provide an even more granular breakdown of component subskills that are either a sequence of developmental precursors or steps in task analyses.

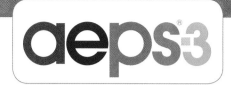

Arrival & Departure

Arrival & Departure includes the activities children participate in when arriving at and departing from a location for caregiving, visiting, socializing, and receiving services such as health care, therapy, and instruction with the intention of interacting and sharing space with others. Children arrive and depart in many ways: being carried, walking, and using riding toys or being pushed in wheelchairs. This routine changes over time as children's motor, adaptive, cognitive, and social-emotional skills increase. Children perform this routine ranging from twice a day to several times a day, depending on how often they enter or exit new environments. The AEPS-3 Beginning level of Arrival & Departure uses skills from six developmental areas.

Concurrent Skills

The following concurrent skills are AEPS-3 skills that can be easily embedded and taught during regular occurrences of Arrival & Departure.

FINE MOTOR Beginning Skills

A 1   Makes directed batting or swiping movements with each hand

A 1.1   Brings hands together near midline

A 2.1   Grasps hand-size object

B 1   Activates object with finger

B 1.1   Uses finger to point or touch

B 1.2   Uses hand to activate object

B 1.3   Uses fingers to explore object

B 2.1   Turns object using either hand

B 3.4   Holds object with one hand and manipulates object or produces action with other hand

B 3.5   Transfers object from hand to hand

D 1.2   Uses finger to interact with touch screen

Embedded Learning Opportunities

- *Brings toys together and transfers from hand to hand while riding in car seat*
- *Points to things (birds, trucks, cars) while riding in car or on bus*
- *Explores clothing with fingers*
- *Holds toy in one hand and uses finger to activate it with other hand*
- *Explores touch screen device in car seat*

GROSS MOTOR Beginning Skills

A 1   Turns head, moves arms, and kicks legs independently of each other

A 1.3   Turns head side to side

A 2   Puts weight on one hand or arm while reaching with opposite hand

A 3   Rolls from back to stomach

A 3.2   Rolls from back or stomach to side

A 4   Assumes balanced sitting position

A 4.1   Assumes hands-and-knees position from sitting

A 4.2   Regains balanced, upright sitting position after reaching across body

A 4.3   Regains balanced, upright sitting position after leaning left, right, and forward

A 4.4   Sits balanced without support

A 4.5   Sits balanced using hands for support

A 4.6   Holds head in midline when sitting supported

A 5   Gets out of chair

A 5.1   Sits down in chair

A 5.2   Maintains sitting position in chair

B 1   Creeps forward using alternating arm and leg movements

B 1.1   Rocks while in creeping position

B 1.2   Assumes creeping position

B 1.3   Crawls forward on stomach

B 1.4   Pivots on stomach

B 2   Stoops and regains balanced standing position

B 2.1   Rises from sitting to standing position

B 2.2   Stands unsupported

B 2.3   Pulls to standing position

B 2.4   Pulls to kneeling position

B 3.1   Walks without support

B 3.2   Walks with one-hand support

B 3.3   Walks with two-hand support

B 3.4   Cruises

C 3.4   Sits on riding toy or in wagon while in motion

Embedded Learning Opportunities

- *Turns head to parent's voice, kicks legs and waves arms at departure from child care*
- *Waves goodbye to adult*
- *Reaches toward adult with one hand while putting weight on other*
- *Rolls from back to stomach or side and sits with or without support while adult dresses child in outerwear*
- *Sits in car seat or wagon with or without support while being pulled to destination*
- *Stands up out of chair after getting shoes on with assistance*
- *Greets adult by rolling over, sitting up, crawling, or getting out of chair and walking to them*
- *Bends down to get shoe and carries it to adult*
- *Stands unsupported while adult puts on jacket*
- *Walks into building with or without support*
- *Cruises down hallway to get to classroom*

SOCIAL-EMOTIONAL　Beginning Skills

A 1　Initiates positive social behavior toward familiar adult

A 1.1　Responds appropriately to familiar adult's affective tone

A 1.2　Responds to familiar adult's positive social behavior

A 2　Maintains social interaction with familiar adult

A 2.1　Initiates simple social interaction with familiar adult

B 2.2　Seeks comfort, closeness, or physical contact from familiar adult

B 2.3　Responds appropriately to soothing by adult

C 1.3　Plays near one or two peers

D 3.3　Entertains self by playing with toys

D 4.2　Claims and defends possessions

Embedded Learning Opportunities

■ *Gives adult hug or kiss upon arrival or departure*

■ *Calms down after separating from caregiver once adult holds and soothes infant*

■ *Crawls to adult to be held*

■ *Holds up foot for sock or shoe while being helped to dress*

■ *Crawls to greet peers upon arrival*

■ *Says "Mine!" when another child tries to take their hat*

SOCIAL-COMMUNICATION　Beginning Skills

A 1　Turns and looks toward person speaking

A 1.1　Quiets to familiar voice

A 2　Produces speech sounds

A 2.1　Coos and gurgles

A 3　Engages in vocal exchanges

A 3.1　Vocalizes to another person expressing positive affective state

A 3.2　Vocalizes to another person expressing negative affective state

A 4　Uses intentional gestures, vocalizations, and objects to communicate

A 4.1　Makes requests of others

A 4.2　Makes choices to express preferences

A 4.3　Expresses desire to continue activity

A 4.4　Expresses negation or protests

B 1　Follows gaze to establish joint attention

B 1.1　Follows pointing gestures with eyes

B 1.2　Looks toward object

B 2.1　Recognizes own and familiar names

B 2.2　Responds to single-word directive

C 1.3　Uses consistent approximations for words or signs

C 1.4　Uses consistent consonant–vowel combinations

Embedded Learning Opportunities

■ *Quiets to familiar voice after being dropped off at child care or school*

■ *Laughs and runs to adult upon departure*

■ *Cries when separating from adult*

■ *Asks for more singing while in car*

■ *Picks up boots to wear instead of shoes*

■ *Looks at adult and points to hat while getting ready*

■ *Points at fire truck and says "fire truck"*

■ *Sees adult's picture and says their name*

■ *Waits by door as asked while adult gets diaper bag*

■ *Says "ba-ba" for bye-bye and waves consistently*

COGNITIVE Beginning Skills

A 1   Orients to events or stimulation

A 1.1   Reacts to events or stimulation

A 2   Combines simple actions to examine people, animals, and objects

A 2.1   Uses sensory means to explore people, animals, and objects

B 1.1   Imitates novel simple motor action not already in repertoire

B 1.2   Imitates familiar simple motor action

B 2.1   Imitates novel vocalizations

B 2.2   Imitates familiar vocalizations

C 1.2   Locates hidden object

D 1.2   Retains one object when second object is obtained

D 2   Coordinates actions with objects to achieve new outcomes

D 2.1   Tries different simple actions to achieve goal

D 2.2   Uses simple actions on objects

E 1.2   Uses senses to explore

E 2.3   Makes observations

Embedded Learning Opportunities

- *Turns head and visually follows others when being dropped off at school or child care*
- *Explores toys by feeling and mouthing while riding in car seat*
- *Waves bye-bye when adult waves upon leaving home or child care program*
- *Imitates familiar vocalizations such as "bye-bye" or "hi"*
- *Locates snack that adult hid in diaper bag*
- *Picks up jacket while still holding shoe*
- *Vocalizes to adult after trying unsuccessfully to reach toy while riding in car*
- *Reaches down and touches wet grass while walking into school*

MATH Beginning Skills

A 1.2   Recites numbers 1–3

Embedded Learning Opportunities

- *Counts "1, 2, 3, in!" [or out] before entering or exiting vehicle*

TIER 1

■ UNIVERSAL STRATEGIES

These are best practices for ALL young children, with attention to meeting learning outcomes within daily routines and activities of family life and early childhood classrooms while promoting positive adult–child relationships and peer interactions.

Arrival and departure in the very early developmental level involve infants and children's increasing independence in motor skills: lying, then sitting and standing to put on and take off outerwear; creeping, crawling, standing, or walking to get to or from the car; sitting supported and later without support in car seats and on riding toys to get to their destinations. As children's cognitive skills develop, they observe and imitate others' actions and imitate vocalizations such as "hi" and "bye-bye" during arrivals and departures. Children begin communicating by establishing joint attention, using consistent signs or word approximations, and responding to familiar names and simple directions. Children interact more with the environment through functional fine motor skills such as pointing, rotating their wrists, transferring objects, and grasping and releasing items during transport.

Interactions

Infants and younger toddlers often experience stress and anxiety upon transitions, especially when changing caregivers. Interactions with adults can provide strong foundations for comfortable transitions when children arrive at and depart from different environments. Following are some suggested interactions for the Beginning level of this routine:

▲ Maintain a cheerful manner (uplifting tone of voice, smiles, encouragement, positive feedback) to help calm young children and prevent stressful transitions.

▲ Keep arrival and departure routines predictable, and allow time to follow children's leads whenever possible.

▲ Promote independence during the routine by allowing children to walk or crawl (safely) to the door.

▲ Take advantage of the opportunities this routine presents to use language to introduce new skills (label objects, use parallel talk to expand on children's vocabulary).

▲ Check arrival and departure environments thoroughly to ensure safety, because this routine includes potential for injury, and use special caution in busy parking lots and crowded hallways.

Environment and Materials

In the earliest developmental stages, during arrival and departure children rely almost totally on adult assistance because of motor limitations and safety concerns. This is so in all environments (home, school, child care, grocery store, relatives' and peers' homes, doctors' offices, and others). The materials and supplies to help ensure smooth arrivals and departures vary from family to family. Some children ride in car seats, whereas others are held or sit on adults' laps on the bus or ride in strollers. Many infants come to recognize the diaper bags adults pack for outings, which may contain arrival and departure items such as outerwear, travel toys, comfort blankets, and snacks.

TIER 2

■ FOCUSED STRATEGIES

These strategies are for teaching SOME children who are struggling with a component of a skill or whose development is stalled and who need extra help to catch up or keep up. The strategies include a variety of minor adaptations or modifications to daily routines, activities, and environments to meet targeted outcomes at home and in classrooms.

▲ Keep arrival and departure routines consistent and predictable. Every time very young children leave or arrive, use the same words and actions and give alerts in advance.

▲ Help adults make transport time a positive and fun experience to help keep children from negatively associating departure and transport with arrival and separation.

▲ Arriving at child care and separating from adults is often more stressful than departing from home.

▲ Have adults say a quick goodbye as they leave, and reassure children about the adults' return. Simultaneously, distract children who are anxious when they arrive by using parallel talk and questions to describe peers, objects, and activities in the room:

△ "I see your favorite truck right here."

△ "Let's see what Alejandro is building in the block area."

△ "Come with me to look out the window at the birds."

▲ Comfort infants who cry after adults leave by carrying them for a few minutes until they calm down enough to engage in play or social activities. At arrival, have musical mobiles, simple noise-making toys, and interactive books available to distract upset and tense young children with engaging activities.

▲ Encourage very young children to use their most sophisticated motor, social, and communication skills independently when arriving and departing:

△ Model saying and waving bye-bye as parents leave.

△ Have children walk to the classroom on their own from outside the door.

▲ Provide simple, one-step directions for children to follow when arriving and departing:

    △ "Wave bye-bye to Daddy."

    △ "Find Mommy by the door."

    △ "Hold my hand."

▲ Offer children multiple opportunities to practice "mini" arrival and departure activities during daily routines:

    △ Have very young children wave bye-bye when leaving the play area for nap.

    △ Say "Time to get our coats on" before going outside.

▲ Have parents bring materials that will ease the transition from one environment to another. Some infants may need a pacifier, and others may need a blanket or stuffed toy from home.

▲ Learn to recognize children's cues and preferences.

▲ Teach children who cannot speak to use simple signs (MORE, ALL DONE) so they can communicate their preferences.

▲ Pair sign language with spoken words for children who are nonverbal or who have hearing impairments.

■ SPECIALIZED STRATEGIES

These strategies for teaching the FEW children who need intensive supports include a variety of specialized, individualized, precise evidence-based strategies to meet children's unique goals/outcomes:

▲ Work with home caregivers to develop specific, consistent procedures for arrival and departure. Update as necessary to address the family's priorities and concerns, and match to young children's changing skills.

▲ Provide desirable, adaptable materials for transport:

    △ Use a wagon, riding toy, or stroller during arrival and departure to take children who cannot walk or crawl to or from their transport to their destination.

▲ Make available to families a "lending library" of specialized equipment for transport and transition, or provide information about community resources for equipment loan.

▲ Work with motor therapists to modify transportation equipment to improve participation and independence for children with specialized fine and gross motor needs.

▲ Teach children who are not yet talking gestures or sign language for greetings and farewells.

▲ Plan gestures and verbal prompts to help children understand what they should be doing during each step of arrival and departure times.

▲ Use sign language with children who have hearing impairments, and be sure to alert them to upcoming transitions.

▲ Describe various environments in detail for children who have vision impairments:

    △ Assign and use a specific name and routine for each destination so children know where they are and what to expect.

    △ Keep aspects of arrival environments as consistent as possible. If changes in child care classrooms are necessary, familiarize infants who have vision impairments with new furniture arrangements, materials, equipment, and supplies in advance.

    △ Introduce new toys and peers individually using touch and sound.

▲ Make sure each destination is accessible to children with specialized physical and communication needs (wheelchair ramps, braille on doors and elevators, wide doors, assistive communication devices).

AEPS-3 Curriculum Resources (Appendix A)

Appendix A in this volume contains numerous additional resources to supplement the AEPS-3 Curriculum. The first part of the appendix presents a list of general curriculum resources, and the second part provides lists of supplementary resources for each individual routine and activity.

AEPS-3 Skills Matrix (Appendix B)

The AEPS-3 Skills Matrix in Appendix B of this volume spotlights individual skills by showing functional application across all routines and activities. Each skills matrix (there are eight total, one for each of the test's eight developmental areas) allows you to select individual AEPS-3 items for children who require an intensive focus on a few skills across routines and activities. For children who have difficulty learning new skills at the level of individual AEPS-3 items, the Foundation Steps (*FS*) provide an even more granular breakdown of component subskills that are either a sequence of developmental precursors or steps in task analyses.

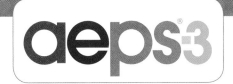

8

Art

Art activities have varying elements that include materials, medium, location, and participants, and they use children's creativity and imagination to create art both indoors and outdoors, at home or in child care settings. Art is not limited to projects that produce permanent products. In early childhood, art is more about the process than the product. This routine changes across skill areas as young children's motor, cognitive, and social skills increase and can address a number of developmental skills depending on the theme. The AEPS-3 Beginning level of Art uses skills from six developmental areas.

Concurrent Skills

The following concurrent skills are AEPS-3 skills that can be easily embedded and taught during regular occurrences of Art.

FINE MOTOR Beginning Skills

A 1   Makes directed batting or swiping movements with each hand

A 1.1   Brings hands together near midline

A 1.2   Makes directed movements with arms

A 2.1   Grasps hand-size object

A 2.2   Grasps small cylindrical object

A 2.4   Grasps hand-size object using whole hand

A 3.1   Releases object into targeted space

A 3.2   Releases object into nondefined space

B 1.1   Uses finger to point or touch

B 1.3   Uses fingers to explore object

B 2.1   Turns object using either hand

B 3.4   Holds object with one hand and manipulates object or produces action with other hand

B 3.5   Transfers object from hand to hand

Embedded Learning Opportunities

- *Swipes hand over paint with each hand*
- *Holds object (jar, playdough container, paint cup) with both hands at midline*
- *Grasps hand-size object (ball, pom-pom)*
- *Grasps markers to do art project*
- *Puts material (crayon, marker, dot marker) away in container (basket, bucket, bag)*
- *Releases material (feather, sticker, pom-pom) onto paper*
- *Releases material (leaf, snowflake, tissue paper) onto wall or window covered with contact paper*
- *Explores paint with finger(s)*
- *Pokes holes in clay or playdough*
- *Holds marker in one hand while attempting to remove marker cap with other hand*
- *Holds paint cup with one hand while painting with other*
- *Transfers playdough from hand to hand*

GROSS MOTOR Beginning Skills

A 4.4   Sits balanced without support

A 4.5   Sits balanced using hands for support

A 4.6   Holds head in midline when sitting supported

A 5   Gets out of chair

A 5.1   Sits down in chair

A 5.2   Maintains sitting position in chair

B 1   Creeps forward using alternating arm and leg movements

B 2   Stoops and regains balanced standing position

B 2.1   Rises from sitting to standing position

B 2.2   Stands unsupported

B 2.3   Pulls to standing position

B 3.1   Walks without support

B 3.2   Walks with one-hand support

B 3.3   Walks with two-hand support

B 3.4   Cruises

Embedded Learning Opportunities

■ *Sits independently while adult shows them art project*

■ *Creeps across floor toward table where art materials are located*

■ *Walks with or without support on paper with paint on feet*

■ *Cruises around table to explore art table activity (playdough, stickers, crayons)*

SOCIAL-EMOTIONAL Beginning Skills

A 1   Initiates positive social behavior toward familiar adult

A 1.1   Responds appropriately to familiar adult's affective tone

A 1.2   Responds to familiar adult's positive social behavior

A 2   Maintains social interaction with familiar adult

A 2.1   Initiates simple social interaction with familiar adult

A 2.2   Repeats part of interactive game or action in order to continue game or action

A 2.3   Responds to familiar game or action

D 3.3   Entertains self by playing with toys

D 4.2   Claims and defends possessions

Embedded Learning Opportunities

■ *Coos while watching adult*

■ *Quiets and listens to adult explain art activity*

■ *Takes turns coloring on paper*

■ *Seeks adult in anticipation of their turn to do art*

■ *Engages with art materials for period of time alone*

■ *Says "Mine!" when another child tries to take art supplies*

SOCIAL-COMMUNICATION Beginning Skills

A 1   Turns and looks toward person speaking

A 1.1   Quiets to familiar voice

A 2   Produces speech sounds

A 2.1   Coos and gurgles

A 3   Engages in vocal exchanges

A 3.1   Vocalizes to another person expressing positive affective state

A 3.2   Vocalizes to another person expressing negative affective state

A 4   Uses intentional gestures, vocalizations, and objects to communicate

A 4.1   Makes requests of others

A 4.2   Makes choices to express preferences

A 4.3   Expresses desire to continue activity

A 4.4   Expresses negation or protests

B 1   Follows gaze to establish joint attention

B 1.1   Follows pointing gestures with eyes

B 1.2   Looks toward object

B 2.1   Recognizes own and familiar names

B 2.2   Responds to single-word directive

C 1.3   Uses consistent approximations for words or signs

C 1.4   Uses consistent consonant–vowel combinations

Embedded Learning Opportunities

■ Quiets and looks at adult explaining art activity

■ Calms when adult says it's time for art

■ Looks at adult and vocalizes speechlike sounds ("ma-ma")

■ Vocalizes (cries, screams, laughs) to adult to express affective state

■ Requests more of material or to continue activity

■ Makes a choice (color to use, materials to use, whether to use brush or hands to paint)

■ Signs or says "more" or "all done" to continue or discontinue an activity

■ Looks toward playdough when adult asks if they want more art materials

■ Responds to own name when adult speaks it and says "Let's paint!"

■ Responds to adult's one-word directions ("wait," "paint," "come")

■ Says "ma" every time they request marker

COGNITIVE Beginning Skills

A 1   Orients to events or stimulation

A 1.1   Reacts to events or stimulation

A 2   Combines simple actions to examine people, animals, and objects

A 2.1   Uses sensory means to explore people, animals, and objects

B 1.1   Imitates novel simple motor action not already in repertoire

B 1.2   Imitates familiar simple motor action

D 1.2   Retains one object when second object is obtained

D 2   Coordinates actions with objects to achieve new outcomes

D 2.1   Tries different simple actions to achieve goal

D 2.2   Uses simple actions on objects

E 1.2   Uses senses to explore

E 2.3   Makes observations

Embedded Learning Opportunities

■ Holds paintbrush and moves arms to paint

■ Explores objects using senses (touches paint, smells playdough)

■ Imitates brush strokes after adult models

■ Touches and smells various art supplies (gak, finger paints, contact paper)

■ Reaches art supplies by climbing on chair after other means of getting to them have been unsuccessful

■ Puts hands in different colored paints and mixes them together to observe colors made

MATH Beginning Skills

A 1.2   Recites numbers 1–3

UNIVERSAL STRATEGIES

These are best practices for ALL young children, with attention to meeting learning outcomes within daily routines and activities of family life and early childhood classrooms while promoting positive adult–child relationships and peer interactions.

Learning art for infants and toddlers at the very earliest levels of development is largely a sensory experience. They can explore objects of different sizes and textures while developing additional fine motor skills, such as grasping small objects, manipulating the objects, and using their fingers to point and touch. As children's cognitive and language skills mature, they become able to coordinate actions, imitate movements, imitate words, and express their preferences. As children's gross motor skills increase, they become able to participate in art by sitting without support (on the floor and in a chair), getting out of a chair, and walking without support.

Interactions

Following are some suggestions to support art routines in the early developmental stages:

▲ Provide developmentally appropriate opportunities for children to experience art both indoors and outdoors throughout each day.

▲ Determine children's likes and dislikes and follow their lead on art projects (unless safety is an issue).

▲ Model art projects for children while using parallel talk to explain what is happening.

▲ Maintain positive interactions with children by smiling and using a pleasant tone of voice, especially when giving specific feedback.

▲ Give young children adequate time to experiment with and explore art materials while encouraging them to observe other children (peers and older) engaging in drawing, painting, coloring, and other art activities.

Environment and Materials

This routine can be implemented both indoors and outdoors. Indoors, children are seated at a table or on the floor to partake in art activities. Outdoors, art activities may take place on a sidewalk, driveway, or any other hard surface such as a child-size picnic table. When completing this routine outside, be aware of heightened safety concerns, such as cars, bicycles, and people walking. Following are some suggestions for environment and materials at the Beginning level:

▲ At times, adults may want to have children walk on paper to create art by putting paint on the bottoms of their feet.

▲ Materials that are needed for art vary on the basis of location and type of art children are creating. Possibilities are nearly endless—many materials can be used in the art routine. Suggestions for indoor art projects are watercolor paints, crayons, finger paints, paint daubers, playdough, clay, colored pencils, and pencils. Other materials may include paper, glue, markers, paper plates, napkins, and paint brushes, to name just a few items. Outside materials include sidewalk chalk, spray bottles, paint, and natural materials (leaves, grass, pine cones). Ensure that whatever products are made available to children are nontoxic for safety reasons, as children at this developmental level tend to put things in their mouths. When possible, use washable materials (paint, markers). Many adults are able to find some type of supplies in their home, so they do not have to purchase them.

■ FOCUSED STRATEGIES

These strategies are for teaching SOME children who are struggling with a component of a skill or whose development is stalled and who need extra help to catch up or keep up. The strategies include a variety of minor adaptations or modifications to daily routines, activities, and environments to meet targeted outcomes at home and in classrooms.

▲ Offer multiple opportunities to repeat the same type of project. Repetition is an important way that children learn one particular art project, which could include using numbers and letters.

▲ Pay close attention for times when infants are comfortable, alert, and ready to learn or play. Children who are tired or uncomfortable may be unwilling to complete any type of artwork.

▲ Use songs to help children remember the steps for painting:

△ Use the tune of a familiar song, such as the hokey pokey, and come up with a song related to painting with watercolors.

▲ Provide longer wait times for a child to start an art project. Some children who have sensory sensitivities may need extra time to get used to the idea that they will stick their hands into something gooey.

▲ Use a verbal prompt and actual object (paintbrush) to alert children when they are transitioning from one activity to another.

▲ Use peer modeling for the art routine. Often, young children will follow the lead of other children before following an adult's lead.

▲ Learn to recognize children's cues and preferences.

▲ Teach children who cannot speak to use simple signs (MORE, ALL DONE) so they can communicate their preferences.

▲ Pair sign language with spoken words for children who are nonverbal or who have hearing impairments.

■ SPECIALIZED STRATEGIES

These strategies for teaching the FEW children who need intensive supports include a variety of specialized, individualized, precise evidence-based strategies to meet children's unique goals/outcomes:

▲ Provide adaptable materials for children to use:

△ Try oversized paintbrushes and jumbo crayons that are easy to hold.

△ Use hook-and-loop fasteners to adapt additional art supplies so children can hold them in their hands.

▲ For children who are unable to speak their wants/needs, support nonverbal participation and selection of preferences:

△ Teach simple signs to use during art activities (MORE, FINISHED).

△ Let the child lead you to their preferred activity.

△ Teach the child to point to their preferred materials.

▲ Use most-to-least prompts so children can complete their art project, providing hand-over-hand and then decreasing support (physical model, direct verbal prompt).

▲ Use tactile or olfactory materials with children who have vision impairments:

  △ Offer gak with uncooked rice in it.

  △ Provide scented markers.

▲ Make sure that children who have physical disabilities are appropriately positioned (hips flexed, feet on floor, chest supported) so that they can use their arms and hands more effectively.

▲ For children who become easily distracted or take extra time to complete an activity, incorporate extra time to complete the project.

▲ Bring materials that will ease the transition from one environment to another. Some infants may need a pacifier, and others may need a blanket.

AEPS-3 Curriculum Resources (Appendix A)

Appendix A in this volume contains numerous additional resources to supplement the AEPS-3 Curriculum. The first part of the appendix presents a list of general curriculum resources, and the second part provides lists of supplementary resources for each individual routine and activity.

AEPS-3 Skills Matrix (Appendix B)

The AEPS-3 Skills Matrix in Appendix B of this volume spotlights individual skills by showing functional application across all routines and activities. Each skills matrix (there are eight total, one for each of the test's eight developmental areas) allows you to select individual AEPS-3 items for children who require an intensive focus on a few skills across routines and activities. For children who have difficulty learning new skills at the level of individual AEPS-3 items, the Foundation Steps (*FS*) provide an even more granular breakdown of component subskills that are either a sequence of developmental precursors or steps in task analyses.

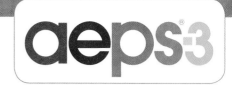

9

Bath Time

Bath Time includes time in the bathtub washing, as well as the skills used before and after bathing. Skills in dressing and undressing can be developed during the bath time routine. The child's participation in this routine increases over time as motor and adaptive skills increase, and they become a more independent participant in all bath time skills. Bath time generally takes place in the child's home, and the occurrence and schedule vary by adult preferences and the child's need for a bath. The AEPS-3 Beginning level of this routine uses skills from seven developmental areas.

Concurrent Skills

The following concurrent skills are AEPS-3 skills that can be easily embedded and taught during regular occurrences of Bath Time.

FINE MOTOR Beginning Skills

A 1 Makes directed batting or swiping movements with each hand

A 1.2 Makes directed movements with arms

A 2.1 Grasps hand-size object

A 3.1 Releases object into targeted space

A 3.2 Releases object into nondefined space

B 2.1 Turns object using either hand

B 3.4 Holds object with one hand and manipulates object or produces action with other hand

Embedded Learning Opportunities

- *Swipes at or bats water to make splash*
- *Holds small bath toy (plastic cup, toy fish, foam numbers and letters)*
- *Drops toy into bathtub to make splash*
- *Turns sponge to "wash" baby in bath*
- *Pulls or pushes plug to fill or drain tub water*
- *Holds empty cup in one hand and second cup full of water in other hand, pours water from full cup into tub*

GROSS MOTOR Beginning Skills

A 1.1 Kicks legs

A 1.2 Waves arms

A 1.3 Turns head side to side

A 4 Assumes balanced sitting position

A 4.2 Regains balanced, upright sitting position after reaching across body

A 4.3 Regains balanced, upright sitting position after leaning left, right, and forward

A 4.4 Sits balanced without support

A 4.5 Sits balanced using hands for support

A 4.6 Holds head in midline when sitting supported

Embedded Learning Opportunities

■ *Kicks legs in tub to make splash*

■ *Turns head from side to side to help wash face and hair*

■ *Sits up straight after leaning forward or to side to reach toy in tub*

■ *Holds head at midline while sitting in tub either without support or with support of bathtub seat*

SOCIAL-EMOTIONAL Beginning Skills

A 1 Initiates positive social behavior toward familiar adult

A 1.1 Responds appropriately to familiar adult's affective tone

A 1.2 Responds to familiar adult's positive social behavior

A 2 Maintains social interaction with familiar adult

A 2.1 Initiates simple social interaction with familiar adult

A 2.2 Repeats part of interactive game or action in order to continue game or action

A 2.3 Responds to familiar game or action

D 3.3 Entertains self by playing with toys

Embedded Learning Opportunities

■ *Smiles at adult singing "Rubber Ducky" to child in tub*

■ *Makes bubble noises while adult makes same noise*

■ *Pulls towel up to cover eyes to keep playing Peekaboo with adult after bath*

■ *Sits in tub and plays with bath toys (cups, toy fish, boats, foam numbers and letters)*

SOCIAL-COMMUNICATION Beginning Skills

A 1   Turns and looks toward person speaking

A 1.1   Quiets to familiar voice

A 2   Produces speech sounds

A 2.1   Coos and gurgles

A 3   Engages in vocal exchanges

A 3.1   Vocalizes to another person expressing positive affective state

A 3.2   Vocalizes to another person expressing negative affective state

A 4   Uses intentional gestures, vocalizations, and objects to communicate

A 4.1   Makes requests of others

A 4.2   Makes choices to express preferences

A 4.3   Expresses desire to continue activity

A 4.4   Expresses negation or protests

B 1   Follows gaze to establish joint attention

B 1.1   Follows pointing gestures with eyes

B 1.2   Looks toward object

B 2.2   Responds to single-word directive

C 1.3   Uses consistent approximations for words or signs

C 1.4   Uses consistent consonant-vowel combinations

Embedded Learning Opportunities

■ *Looks toward adult and quiets when adult says "Time for a bath"*

■ *Coos or vocalizes to adult who is talking during bath*

■ *Points and vocalizes to gain adult's attention to indicate desire for bath toys*

■ *Shrugs shoulder to indicate wish to have more water poured on self*

■ *Cries or moves away from tub to indicate wish not to take bath*

■ *Looks at plastic bath book when adult points to picture and labels it*

■ *Sits down in tub or sink when adult says "Time to sit down!"*

COGNITIVE Beginning Skills

A 1   Orients to events or stimulation

A 1.1   Reacts to events or stimulation

A 2   Combines simple actions to examine people, animals, and objects

A 2.1   Uses sensory means to explore people, animals, and objects

B 1.1   Imitates novel simple motor action not already in repertoire

B 1.2   Imitates familiar simple motor action

B 2.1   Imitates novel vocalizations

B 2.2   Imitates familiar vocalizations

C 1.2   Locates hidden object

D 1.1   Uses part of object or support to obtain another object

D 1.2   Retains one object when second object is obtained

D 2   Coordinates actions with objects to achieve new outcomes

D 2.1   Tries different simple actions to achieve goal

E 1.2   Uses senses to explore

E 2.3   Makes observations

Embedded Learning Opportunities

■ *Turns head toward adult and smiles when adult pours water on child's back*

■ *Says "Vroom, vroom" when pushing boat in tub after adult models sound*

■ *Finds bath toy under plastic cup after adult hides it*

LITERACY Beginning Skills

A 1.1 Participates in shared one-on-one reading

Embedded Learning Opportunities

■ *Labels or identifies pictures for adult while reading in tub*

MATH Beginning Skills

A 1.2 Recites numbers 1–3

Embedded Learning Opportunities

■ *Repeats "1, 2, 3" after adult says "1, 2, 3, up!" when lifting child out of tub*

TIER 1

■ UNIVERSAL STRATEGIES

These are best practices for ALL young children, with attention to meeting learning outcomes within daily routines and activities of family life and early childhood classrooms while promoting positive adult–child relationships and peer interactions.

At the Beginning level, an adult must carry out the bath time routine because the adaptive skills children need for this routine are not yet developed. For safety reasons, it is essential for the adult to remain present during all parts of the routine. The adult must decide when a bath is necessary and make preparations so the routine is as predictable and enjoyable as possible for infants or young toddlers. Repetition (always washing body parts in the same order, giving the bath at approximately the same time every time) is an easy way to make the routine comfortable and predictable. Cognitive, math, literacy, and social-communication skills can be developed during bath time by providing a variety of age-appropriate toys that are suitable for use in water.

Interactions

It is most important to make sure bath time is a safe, positive experience for children. Following are some suggested interactions for the Beginning level of this routine:

▲ Describe aloud what is happening during each part of the bathing routine ("I am going to wash your hair now").

▲ Sing songs or play silly games not only to help make bath time a positive experience but also to teach names of body parts.

▲ Encourage children to participate actively in bath time as they get older, to develop adaptive skills such as dressing and undressing and washing independently.

▲ Model how to push a boat in the water while making a "vroom" sound.

▲ Let children take a bath book into the tub to look at with an adult and label the pictures.

▲ Help children line up foam numbers on the side of the tub and count them.

▲ Spell out the child's name with foam letters on the side of the tub.

Environment/Materials

The bath place may include an infant-size bathtub or regular-size tub with a bath seat for children who need support to sit up, and in some cases, it may also include a sink. Materials needed typically include soap, shampoo, washcloth, towel, diaper, robe or clothing, and toys.

Following are some suggestions for environment and materials at the Beginning level of this routine:

▲ Keep on hand bath-safe toys (bath books, stackable cups, foam letters and numbers of all shapes and sizes) to encourage children to manipulate and explore different items.

▲ Consider using regular household items (unbreakable drinking cups, measuring cups, spoons) as appropriate bath toys.

▲ Make sure all materials needed for bath time are easily accessible next to the bathing area <u>before</u> putting a child in the bathwater. Never leave a child alone to get materials for a bath.

▲ Read books with a bath time routine in them to help prepare children for their own bath (*Five Little Monkeys Jumping in the Bath,* Christelow, 2012).

■ FOCUSED STRATEGIES

These strategies are for teaching SOME children who are struggling with a component of a skill or whose development is stalled and who need extra help to catch up or keep up. The strategies include a variety of minor adaptations or modifications to daily routines, activities, and environments to meet targeted outcomes at home and in classrooms.

▲ Use small amounts of water in the bathtub if children show fear of water.

▲ Let children touch the water in the tub before placing them in it. This may help reassure children who are uneasy about the sensory experience of being in water.

▲ Ask children to place bath toys in the tub before putting them in it. Giving children some control and choice in ways like this can help make the experience more enjoyable.

▲ Use a visual timer to alert children when bath time begins and ends.

▲ Accommodate children's sensory concerns by using clothing and towels in fabrics they prefer.

▲ Learn to recognize children's cues and preferences.

▲ Teach children who cannot speak to use simple signs (MORE, ALL DONE) so they can communicate their preferences.

▲ Pair sign language with spoken words for children who are nonverbal or who have hearing impairments.

■ SPECIALIZED STRATEGIES

These strategies for teaching the FEW children who need intensive supports include a variety of specialized, individualized, precise evidence-based strategies to meet children's unique goals/outcomes:

▲ Adapt the routine for children on the basis of their physical abilities:

△ Use a specialized bath seat to provide support and some independence for children who are unable to sit up.

▲ Use positive reinforcement to increase children's willingness to participate in bath time:

△ Allow children to choose an additional book to read at the end of the routine as a reward.

▲ Use naturalistic language prompting strategies such as mand modeling (see Chapter 4) to encourage children to ask for what they want and to minimize protests:

△ Ask the child what they want to do during bathing.

△ Model saying "more" (to encourage the child to request what they want more of, such as splashing) or "all done" (to encourage the child to say when they want to refuse something or are finished, such as when they wish to get out of the tub).

△ Ask what the child wants and wait for them to respond by signing or using a word to say "more" or "all done."

△ If the child does not do so, provide verbal directions or offer a physical model to show them what to do or say, and then give them an opportunity to make the request.

AEPS-3 Curriculum Resources (Appendix A)

Appendix A in this volume contains numerous additional resources to supplement the AEPS-3 Curriculum. The first part of the appendix presents a list of general curriculum resources, and the second part provides lists of supplementary resources for each individual routine and activity.

AEPS-3 Skills Matrix (Appendix B)

The AEPS-3 Skills Matrix in Appendix B of this volume spotlights individual skills by showing functional application across all routines and activities. Each skills matrix (there are eight total, one for each of the test's eight developmental areas) allows you to select individual AEPS-3 items for children who require an intensive focus on a few skills across routines and activities. For children who have difficulty learning new skills at the level of individual AEPS-3 items, the Foundation Steps (FS) provide an even more granular breakdown of component subskills that are either a sequence of developmental precursors or steps in task analyses.

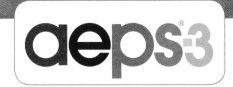

10

Block Play

Block Play consists of playing with blocks made from different materials, in a variety of shapes, sizes, and colors. This activity may also include other toys to combine with block play (cars, people, animals). Children's participation in block play changes over time as fine motor and cognitive skills increase and play becomes more purposeful and active. This activity can take place at home or in child care settings and may occur several times a day depending on children's interest level and schedule. The AEPS-3 Beginning level of Block Play covers six developmental areas.

Concurrent Skills

The concurrent skills below are AEPS-3 skills that can be easily embedded and taught during regular occurrences of Block Play.

FINE MOTOR Beginning Skills

A 1   Makes directed batting or swiping movements with each hand

A 1.1   Brings hands together near midline

A 1.2   Makes directed movements with arms

A 2.1   Grasps hand-size object

A 2.2   Grasps small cylindrical object

A 2.4   Grasps hand-size object using whole hand

A 3   Stacks objects

A 3.1   Releases object into targeted space

A 3.2   Releases object into nondefined space

B 1.1   Uses finger to point or touch

B 1.3   Uses fingers to explore object

B 2.1   Turns object using either hand

B 3.4   Holds object with one hand and manipulates object or produces action with other hand

B 3.5   Transfers object from hand to hand

Embedded Learning Opportunities

- *Knocks down soft block tower by batting at it*

- *Holds one block in each hand and bangs them together*

- *Grasps blocks of different shapes (rectangular, cylindrical, triangular)*

- *Drops block or toy onto a targeted space (another block, car, animal)*

- *Builds block tower*

- *Releases block or toy into large bin or basket*

- *Pokes block towers to knock down*

- *Uses fingers to explore materials (blocks, people, animals)*

- *Turns parts of toy with either hand*

- *Holds toy in one hand while pushing car with other hand*

- *Moves block from one hand to other*

■ 71

GROSS MOTOR Beginning Skills

A 1   Turns head, moves arms, and kicks legs independently of each other

A 1.1   Kicks legs

A 1.2   Waves arms

A 1.3   Turns head side to side

A 2   Puts weight on one hand or arm while reaching with opposite hand

A 2.1   Remains propped on extended arms with head lifted

A 2.2   Remains propped on nonextended forearms with head lifted

A 3   Rolls from back to stomach

A 3.1   Rolls from stomach to back

A 3.2   Rolls from back or stomach to side

A 4   Assumes balanced sitting position

A 4.1   Assumes hands-and-knees position from sitting

A 4.2   Regains balanced, upright sitting position after reaching across body

A 4.3   Regains balanced, upright sitting position after leaning left, right, and forward

A 4.4   Sits balanced without support

A 4.5   Sits balanced using hands for support

A 4.6   Holds head in midline when sitting supported

B 1   Creeps forward using alternating arm and leg movements

B 1.1   Rocks while in creeping position

B 1.2   Assumes creeping position

B 1.3   Crawls forward on stomach

B 1.4   Pivots on stomach

B 2   Stoops and regains balanced standing position

B 2.1   Rises from sitting to standing position

B 2.2   Stands unsupported

B 2.3   Pulls to standing position

B 2.4   Pulls to kneeling position

B 3.1   Walks without support

B 3.2   Walks with one-hand support

B 3.3   Walks with two-hand support

B 3.4   Cruises

C 1.6   Throws or rolls ball at target with two hands

Embedded Learning Opportunities

■ *Lies on floor, waves arms, kicks at toys*

■ *Reaches for block with one arm while putting weight on other arm*

■ *Props self on one arm while on stomach and reaches for blocks with other arm*

■ *Rolls to explore toys in block area*

■ *Sits balanced with or without support while playing*

■ *Creeps or crawls to get more blocks or toys*

■ *Crawls forward to get blocks out of reach*

■ *Remains on stomach while pivoting to reach more blocks*

■ *Uses both hands to throw ball at block tower built by adult*

SOCIAL-EMOTIONAL Beginning Skills

A 1   Initiates positive social behavior toward familiar adult

A 1.1   Responds appropriately to familiar adult's affective tone

A 1.2   Responds to familiar adult's positive social behavior

A 2   Maintains social interaction with familiar adult

A 2.1   Initiates simple social interaction with familiar adult

A 2.2   Repeats part of interactive game or action in order to continue game or action

A 2.3   Responds to familiar game or action

B 2.2   Seeks comfort, closeness, or physical contact from familiar adult

B 2.3   Responds appropriately to soothing by adult

C 1.3   Plays near one or two peers

D 3.3   Entertains self by playing with toys

D 4.2   Claims and defends possessions

Embedded Learning Opportunities

- *Gives adult a hug or kiss*
- *Repeats "Knock over block game!"*
- *Runs to adult when adult starts stacking blocks*
- *Sits in adult's lap when stranger enters room*
- *Plays with blocks near one or two peers*
- *Plays alone with cars and blocks*
- *Says "Mine!" when another child tries to take toy*

SOCIAL-COMMUNICATION Beginning Skills

A 1   Turns and looks toward person speaking

A 1.1   Quiets to familiar voice

A 2   Produces speech sounds

A 2.1   Coos and gurgles

A 3   Engages in vocal exchanges

A 3.1   Vocalizes to another person expressing positive affective state

A 3.2   Vocalizes to another person expressing negative affective state

A 4   Uses intentional gestures, vocalizations, and objects to communicate

A 4.1   Makes requests of others

A 4.2   Makes choices to express preferences

A 4.3   Expresses desire to continue activity

A 4.4   Expresses negation or protests

B 1   Follows gaze to establish joint attention

B 1.1   Follows pointing gestures with eyes

B 1.2   Looks toward object

B 2.1   Recognizes own and familiar names

B 2.2   Responds to single-word directive

C 1.3   Uses consistent approximations for words or signs

C 1.4   Uses consistent consonant-vowel combinations

Embedded Learning Opportunities

- *Quiets on hearing familiar voice when fussing*
- *Cries or screams when another child knocks down block tower*
- *Requests more blocks by using sign language*
- *Says "All done" when finished playing with blocks*
- *Finds horse in animal basket when adult asks, "Where's the horse?"*
- *Stops throwing blocks when adult says "Stop!"*
- *Says "ca" every time to label a car*

COGNITIVE Beginning Skills

A 1	Orients to events or stimulation
A 1.1	Reacts to events or stimulation
A 2	Combines simple actions to examine people, animals, and objects
A 2.1	Uses sensory means to explore people, animals, and objects
B 1.1	Imitates novel simple motor action not already in repertoire
B 1.2	Imitates familiar simple motor action
B 2.1	Imitates novel vocalizations
B 2.2	Imitates familiar vocalizations
C 1.2	Locates hidden object
D 1	Uses object to obtain another object
D 1.1	Uses part of object or support to obtain another object
D 1.2	Retains one object when second object is obtained
D 2	Coordinates actions with objects to achieve new outcomes
D 2.1	Tries different simple actions to achieve goal
D 2.2	Uses simple actions on objects
E 1.2	Uses senses to explore
E 2.3	Makes observations

Embedded Learning Opportunities

- *Looks at adult and smiles when adult initiates block play*
- *Turns head in direction of blocks that fell over and made noise*
- *Mouths and feels different types of blocks*
- *Imitates adult stacking and knocking blocks over*
- *Uses one block to pull another block closer*
- *Says "Boom!" after adult says "1, 2, 3, boom!" and knocks down block tower*
- *Locates blocks under blanket after seeing adult hide them*
- *Moves blocks around to achieve stable tower*
- *Dumps basket of blocks to find certain kind after digging through basket*

MATH Beginning Skills

A 1.2 Recites numbers 1-3

Embedded Learning Opportunities

- *Counts "1, 2, 3!" before knocking over block tower*

◼ UNIVERSAL STRATEGIES

These are best practices for ALL young children, with attention to meeting learning outcomes within daily routines and activities of family life and early childhood classrooms while promoting positive adult–child relationships and peer interactions.

Block play for infants and children at the Beginning level involves using fine motor skills to grasp, stack, and bring blocks to the midline of the body to bang together, along with purposefully releasing the blocks into both targeted and nontargeted spaces. As gross motor skills increase, children are able to sit with and without support to play with blocks, cruise to the blocks area, and begin to walk to and from the block area. Cognitively, they use their senses to explore the blocks, imitate motor actions of peers and adults, and attempt different actions to achieve a goal, such as building a tower. Socially, children start to communicate by making requests of others using consistent signs or word approximations, entertaining themselves with the blocks, and claiming and defending their block creations when others are near.

Interactions

At the Beginning level, adults can support block play by providing developmentally appropriate opportunities for children to experience playing with blocks both indoors and outdoors throughout each day. Following are some suggested interactions for the Beginning level:

▲ Model stacking blocks while introducing new words for colors, numbers, and shapes, using a calm, relaxed tone of voice.

▲ Introduce concepts and words such as *big, little, up, down, over,* and *under.*

▲ Allow children time to build a tower or bridge themselves before helping them, giving them a chance to verbally ask for help if they do need it.

▲ Model using additional toys to play with the blocks, using parallel talk to make sure children know what is happening.

▲ Teach the child they may knock over their own blocks while playing by using their hands or other objects, but they may not knock over or break others' block creations.

▲ Follow children's leads and interests during block play:

△ If a child wants to build a man, let them do so, and keep using parallel talk to explain what the child is doing. At this age, children may not verbalize much, but they are listening to everything adults say.

△ Incorporate math into block play by counting "1, 2, 3" before crashing a toy car into the blocks or throwing a ball at the blocks.

Environment and Materials

Block play can take place indoors, outdoors, at home, or at child care, depending on preference. Particularly if block play occurs outside, adults must ensure that the area is safe for infant play. Following are some suggestions for environment and materials at the Beginning level:

▲ Provide buckets of blocks of different shapes, sizes, and colors, made from different materials (foam, wood, plastic, cardboard). Blocks may be store-bought or handmade.

▲ Include other items that complement block play, such as toy cars, animals, people, balls, blankets, baskets, and pails.

▲ Refrain from using any materials that could pose a choking hazard.

▲ Ensure safety with materials used because young children like to put things in their mouth and chew on them:

△ Make sure the paint used on any handmade blocks is nontoxic.

△ Keep block size in mind.

TIER 2

■ FOCUSED STRATEGIES

These strategies are for teaching SOME children who are struggling with a component of a skill or whose development is stalled and who need extra help to catch up or keep up. The strategies include a variety of minor adaptations or modifications to daily routines, activities, and environments to meet targeted outcomes at home and in classrooms.

▲ Follow children's lead. If they need to take a break from blocks, do a different activity for a while and revisit the blocks later to work on skills.

▲ Notice when children are comfortable, alert, and ready to play to promote successful block play. Children who are tired, uncomfortable, or hungry may be unwilling to sit, crawl, or pick up blocks to play.

▲ Simplify activities during block play:

  △ Show children one activity to do with the blocks, such as building a tower, and limit the number of blocks provided to avoid overstimulation.

▲ Allow children to knock over an adult's tower while the adult models and verbally talks about their feelings ("This is fun!"; "You can knock over your tower now"). Never knock over a child's tower without their permission.

▲ Provide verbal prompts to encourage children to build a tower.

▲ Use verbal prompts and real objects to help infants understand transitions.

▲ Use consistent language when talking with children about the routine.

▲ If children are unable to communicate verbally, teach them simple signs related to block play (MORE, HELP).

▲ Vary the environments where block play occurs (indoors, outdoors, tabletop, floor) so children can practice their skills, using settings children find interesting.

▲ Teach children who cannot speak to use simple signs (MORE, ALL DONE).

▲ Pair sign language with spoken words for students who are nonverbal or who have hearing impairments.

▲ Learn to recognize children's cues and preferences.

◼ SPECIALIZED STRATEGIES

These strategies for teaching the FEW children who need intensive supports include a variety of specialized, individualized, precise evidence-based strategies to meet children's unique goals/outcomes:

▲ Adapt the routine for children based on their physical and cognitive abilities:

  △ Carry children who cannot walk or crawl to the block area.

  △ Bring blocks to children if necessary.

▲ Provide adaptable materials:

  △ Use an infant seat or highchair for children who are unable to sit upright on the floor.

▲ Accept nonverbal communication for children who are unable to speak their preferences (moving in the direction of block activity, turning away from blocks when finished).

▲ Use verbal prompts paired with models to help children understand what to do during block play.

▲ Use graduated guidance with hand-over-hand support to help children build and play as needed (see Chapter 4).

▲ Use tactile materials and describe toys verbally to children who have impaired vision.

▲ Adapt blocks so all children can hold them:

  △ Provide blocks of different sizes.

  △ Use soft blocks that can easily fit into children's hands.

▲ Make sure children with physical disabilities are positioned appropriately (hips flexed, feet on floor, chest supported) so they can use their arms and hands to play with blocks more comfortably and effectively.

AEPS-3 Curriculum Resources (Appendix A)

Appendix A in this volume contains numerous additional resources to supplement the AEPS-3 Curriculum. The first part of the appendix presents a list of general curriculum resources, and the second part provides lists of supplementary resources for each individual routine and activity.

AEPS-3 Skills Matrix (Appendix B)

The AEPS-3 Skills Matrix in Appendix B of this volume spotlights individual skills by showing functional application across all routines and activities. Each skills matrix (there are eight total, one for each of the test's eight developmental areas) allows you to select individual AEPS-3 items for children who require an intensive focus on a few skills across routines and activities. For children who have difficulty learning new skills at the level of individual AEPS-3 items, the Foundation Steps (*FS*) provide an even more granular breakdown of component subskills that are either a sequence of developmental precursors or steps in task analyses.

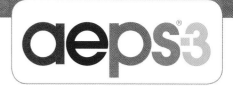

11

Circle Time

Circle Time incorporates many skills and activities, including storytime (looking at and reading books), singing with others, rhyming, identifying letters, reading a class schedule, and choosing activities, among numerous others. This routine changes over time as children's social-communication, social-emotional, cognitive, and literacy skills become more advanced. Circle time occurs most commonly in a classroom or child care setting, and storytime may occur in any setting with an adult or other person with whom a child can share books. Depending on the environment and the schedule, this activity may occur up to three times a day. The AEPS-3 Beginning level of Circle Time includes skills from seven developmental areas.

Concurrent Skills

The following concurrent skills are AEPS-3 skills that can be easily embedded and taught during regular occurrences of Circle Time.

FINE MOTOR Beginning Skills

A 1.1   Brings hands together near midline

A 1.2   Makes directed movements with arms

A 2   Grasps pea-sized object

A 2.1   Grasps hand-sized object

A 3.1   Releases object into targeted space

B 1.1   Uses finger to point or touch

B 2.1   Turns object using either hand

Embedded Learning Opportunities

- *Claps hands during song*
- *Grasps hand-size plastic egg filled with beans and uses as shaker*
- *Places small object (finger puppet, toy animal, instrument) back in adult's hand after song*
- *Puts small object back in basket*
- *Points to pictures in book*
- *Turns shaker over in hand to cause it to make noise*

GROSS MOTOR Beginning Skills

A 4   Assumes balanced sitting position

A 4.1 Assumes hands-and-knees position from sitting

A 4.2 Regains balanced, upright sitting position after reaching across body

A 4.3 Regains balanced, upright sitting position after leaning left, right, and forward

A 4.4 Sits balanced without support

A 4.5 Sits balanced using hands for support

A 4.6 Holds head in midline when sitting supported

B 2   Stoops and regains balanced standing position

B 2.1 Rises from sitting to standing position

B 3.1 Walks without support

B 3.2 Walks with one-hand support

B 3.3 Walks with two-hand support

Embedded Learning Opportunities

■ *Sits balanced with or without support during storytime*

■ *Imitates adult and gets on hands and knees during movement song (pretends to be dog or cat and crawls around room)*

■ *Bends down to pick up object (scarf, instrument) and stands back up during movement song*

■ *Walks with or without support to move around circle during movement activity*

■ *Follows teacher's modeling of movement (yoga, dancing, stretching, rising from sitting to standing)*

SOCIAL-EMOTIONAL Beginning Skills

A 1   Initiates positive social behavior toward familiar adult

A 1.1 Responds appropriately to familiar adult's affective tone

A 1.2 Responds to familiar adult's positive social behavior

A 2.2 Repeats part of interactive game or action in order to continue game or action

A 2.3 Responds to familiar game or action

B 2.2 Seeks comfort, closeness, or physical contact from familiar adult

Embedded Learning Opportunities

■ *Coos while adult sings*

■ *Calms and stops crying when adult starts singing*

■ *Starts clapping hands when song involves clapping ("Pat-a-cake," "If You're Happy and You Know It")*

■ *Asks for music after welcome song*

■ *Sits in adult's lap for story*

SOCIAL-COMMUNICATION Beginning Skills

A 1 Turns and looks toward person speaking

A 1.1 Quiets to familiar voice

A 2 Produces speech sounds

A 2.1 Coos and gurgles

A 3 Engages in vocal exchanges

A 3.1 Vocalizes to another person expressing positive affective state

A 3.2 Vocalizes to another person expressing negative affective state

A 4 Uses intentional gestures, vocalizations, and objects to communicate

A 4.1 Makes requests of others

A 4.2 Makes choices to express preferences

A 4.3 Expresses desire to continue activity

A 4.4 Expresses negation or protests

B 1 Follows gaze to establish joint attention

B 1.1 Follows pointing gestures with eyes

B 1.2 Looks toward object

B 2.1 Recognizes own and familiar names

B 2.2 Responds to single-word directive

C 1.3 Uses consistent approximations for words or signs

C 1.4 Uses consistent consonant–vowel combinations

Embedded Learning Opportunities

- *Turns toward adult reading story*

- *Stops crying once adult starts singing song*

- *Produces prolonged vowel sounds in singsong manner ("aaaaa-aaaaa")*

- *Signs or says "more" or "all done" to voice preference while adult sings songs*

- *Chooses between two colored scarves or two instruments for dancing*

- *Looks at or points to familiar people or pets in family pictures when adult prompts with question (adult asks, "Where's mama?" and child points to picture of mother)*

- *Points to storybook they want adult to read*

- *Sits down when adult says to do so during circle time*

- *Says or signs "more" to tell adult they want to sing more songs or read more books*

COGNITIVE Beginning Skills

A 1   Orients to events or stimulation

A 1.1   Reacts to events or stimulation

A 2   Combines simple actions to examine people, animals, and objects

A 2.1   Uses sensory means to explore people, animals, and objects

B 1.1   Imitates novel simple motor action not already in repertoire

B 1.2   Imitates familiar simple motor action

B 2.1   Imitates novel vocalizations

B 2.2   Imitates familiar vocalizations

E 1.2   Uses senses to explore

E 2.3   Makes observations

Embedded Learning Opportunities

- *Looks at adult after adult starts reading or singing*
- *Looks at adult when adult uses object to make sound (tambourine, shaker)*
- *Laughs or smiles when adult uses object to gain attention (uses puppet to sing song, uses drum while singing song)*
- *Holds and explores tangible object (puppet, small toy, instrument)*
- *Imitates clapping hands, waving, patting knees, other simple motor actions*
- *Says "moo" after adult says "moo" during song, says "car" after adult reads book about cars*
- *Shakes instrument to hear its sound*

LITERACY Beginning Skills

A 1.1   Participates in shared one-on-one reading

Embedded Learning Opportunities

- *Sits in adult's lap to listen to story*

MATH Beginning Skills

A 1.2   Recites numbers 1–3

Embedded Learning Opportunities

- *Recites numbers as adult reads counting book*
- *Counts to three to reveal surprise (puppet, new book, new song)*

TIER 1

■ UNIVERSAL STRATEGIES

These are best practices for ALL young children, with attention to meeting learning outcomes within daily routines and activities of family life and early childhood classrooms while promoting positive adult–child relationships and peer interactions.

Infants and children at the Beginning level are dependent on adults to help them carry out the circle time routine. Cognitively, children develop skills to imitate new words, vocalizations, and motor actions they observe others doing. As social skills develop, they become able to make requests, express their preferences about continuing or discontinuing activities, and initiate familiar activities such as grabbing a favorite book for storytime. Children may listen to stories one to one, label and point to familiar people and objects in picture books, and gain the awareness that pictures represent text. Motor skills also develop during circle time. When planning the routine, apply these best practices:

▲ Consider choosing a welcome song to signal that circle time is about to begin, so children will come join the circle if they desire.

▲ Make sure the environment includes alternative developmentally appropriate activities for children who choose not to join the circle.

▲ Keep in mind that children at this age may be able to sit for only short amounts of time. Include short books or stories, movements, songs, or fingerplay.

▲ Invite children to dance to movement songs or clap to a familiar song.

Interactions

At the Beginning level, adults can support circle time skills by providing opportunities for children to experience the routine throughout the day. Circle time activities might include songs, movement, and literacy activities such as reading books. Children at this developmental stage most often make choices by pointing at their choice or using their whole hand to touch it. Children are most likely to enjoy circle time when they are well rested and are not hungry. Following are some suggestions for interactions at the Beginning level:

▲ Consider including activities such as singing a song about who is at school or child care today, listening to the teacher tell a story with a puppet or prop, and dancing to a fun song.

▲ Watch closely for times when infants are comfortable, alert, and ready to learn or play, as they are most likely to participate in activities actively at these times.

▲ Start teaching expectations around listening during circle time through repetition and consistency.

▲ Follow children's lead. For example, if children move in the direction of a particular instrument, such as piano mats, drums, or shakers, engage the child with that instrument.

▲ Give children choices whenever possible. For example, when choosing a book to read,

  △ Present two options the child may choose between.

  △ Ask "Do you want to read this book [say the book's title and move the book closer to the child] or this book [say the second book's title, and move that book closer while moving the first book farther away]?"

▲ While reading, point to words and pictures to help children understand the relationship between the words and pictures and the text.

▲ Take the time to read to children anytime they want to do so.

Environment and Materials

Circle time most often takes place indoors in one location in a child care, school, or home setting. With appropriate materials and weather permitting, this routine can also occur outdoors. Materials needed include books on various topics that interest children. A rug to sit on can also be a good visual prompt to show children where they need to be located for the routine. Following are some suggestions for environment and materials at the Beginning level:

▲ Ensure safety by keeping the circle time area clean and free of items that might pose a tripping hazard.

▲ Have materials set up and ready for this routine so children do not have to wait.

▲ When choosing books to have on hand for circle time, consider including the following:

△ Short books, because many young children have not yet developed a long attention span

△ Sensory (touch and feel) books, picture books, and books with a few words or sentences on each page

△ Board books—the preferred type for children at the Beginning level, because board books are sturdy and can withstand young children's handling and mouthing them

▲ Incorporate puppets and tangible objects into the routine to encourage children to participate and stay interested (an adult singing "Old McDonald" might also hand each child a small toy farm animal).

▲ Use felt storyboards to help visual learners follow a story.

▲ Keep a music player on hand to play music children can dance to.

■ FOCUSED STRATEGIES

TIER 2

These strategies are for teaching SOME children who are struggling with a component of a skill or whose development is stalled and who need extra help to catch up or keep up. The strategies include a variety of minor adaptations or modifications to daily routines, activities, and environments to meet targeted outcomes at home and in classrooms.

▲ Offer multiple opportunities to read throughout the day. Children may need one-to-one reading instead of a group setting.

▲ Shorten the routine to help support children who can sit for only a minute or two.

▲ Read the same book several times, because repetition is an effective way to expand children's language and understanding of content.

▲ Tailor circles to small group interests, planning two separate circle times if necessary (some children may be interested in the routine only when it focuses on a topic they like, such as cars, animals, or food).

▲ Group children in ways that help eliminate behavior issues.

▲ Use the fact that children love to observe novel actions to help capture and hold their attention during circle time:

△ Use songs and fingerplay to gain infants' attention.

△ Use props (musical instruments, puppets, scarves).

△ Vary tone of voice and volume (whisper songs that are usually sung loudly, slow down to emphasize a word).

▲ Sing a song with one child to help encourage others to join in.

▲ Model desired behaviors and language for children.

▲ Seat assistants beside children who may need extra help during circle time.

▲ Learn to recognize children's cues and preferences.

▲ Teach children who cannot speak to use simple signs (MORE, ALL DONE) so they can communicate their preferences.

▲ Pair sign language with spoken words for students who are nonverbal or who have hearing impairments.

■ SPECIALIZED STRATEGIES

These strategies for teaching the FEW children who need intensive supports include a variety of specialized, individualized, precise evidence-based strategies to meet children's unique goals/outcomes:

▲ Have an adult hold the child or use a support pillow or seat to help children who cannot sit independently.

▲ Give multiple verbal prompts for transitions, and talk children through transitions in a comforting way:

　△ Use songs to signal time for a transition.

　△ Bring materials that help ease transitions (pacifier, chewie, blanket) from one environment to another.

▲ Use hand-under-hand assistance to help children with visual impairments do hand movements to music.

▲ Provide tangibles related to the story (dolls, realistic toy animals, instruments) to hold for children who have visual or hearing impairments; have an adult sit with them and explain the objects while the story is read aloud.

AEPS-3 Curriculum Resources (Appendix A)

Appendix A in this volume contains numerous additional resources to supplement the AEPS-3 Curriculum. The first part of the appendix presents a list of general curriculum resources, and the second part provides lists of supplementary resources for each individual routine and activity.

AEPS-3 Skills Matrix (Appendix B)

The AEPS-3 Skills Matrix in Appendix B of this volume spotlights individual skills by showing functional application across all routines and activities. Each skills matrix (there are eight total, one for each of the test's eight developmental areas) allows you to select individual AEPS-3 items for children who require an intensive focus on a few skills across routines and activities. For children who have difficulty learning new skills at the level of individual AEPS-3 items, the Foundation Steps (*FS*) provide an even more granular breakdown of component subskills that are either a sequence of developmental precursors or steps in task analyses.

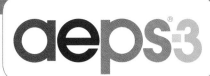

12

Diapering, Toileting, & Handwashing

Diapering, Toileting, & Handwashing includes becoming independent in completing the component tasks that comprise this routine, as well as getting to and from the bathroom or changing location, getting on the toilet, and getting up to the sink. This routine changes significantly over time as children's motor and adaptive skills increase and they begin to take greater interest in completing tasks independently. This routine takes place in all environments, including school, home, child care, and community facilities. The AEPS-3 Beginning level of this routine uses skills from six developmental areas.

Concurrent Skills

The following concurrent skills are AEPS-3 skills that can be easily embedded and taught during regular occurrences of Diapering, Toileting, & Handwashing.

FINE MOTOR Beginning Skills

A 1   Makes directed batting or swiping movements with each hand

A 1.1 Brings hands together near midline

A 1.2 Makes directed movements with arms

A 2   Grasps pea-sized object

A 2.1 Grasps hand-sized object

B 1   Activates object with finger

B 2.1 Turns object using either hand

B 3.5 Transfers object from hand to hand

Embedded Learning Opportunities

- *Uses hand to hit at mobile placed above diaper changing area*

- *Claps in response to adult's saying "Yay, we're all finished!"*

- *Grasps and turns toy during diaper changing*

- *Pushes soap dispenser with single finger*

- *Holds clean diaper in one hand and transfers it to other before handing it to adult*

■ 87

GROSS MOTOR Beginning Skills

A 1   Turns head, moves arms, and kicks legs
       independently of each other

A 1.1 Kicks legs

B 3.1 Walks without support

B 3.2 Walks with one-hand support

B 3.3 Walks with two-hand support

Embedded Learning Opportunities

■ *Kicks legs during diaper change to express excitement or discontent*

■ *Walks to diaper changing area with or without support*

SOCIAL-EMOTIONAL Beginning Skills

A 1   Initiates positive social behavior toward familiar adult

A 1.1 Responds appropriately to familiar adult's affective tone

A 1.2 Responds to familiar adult's positive social behavior

A 2   Maintains social interaction with familiar adult

A 2.1 Initiates social interaction with familiar adult

B 2.2 Seeks comfort, closeness, or physical contact from familiar adult

B 2.3 Responds appropriately to soothing by adult

Embedded Learning Opportunities

■ *Covers eyes while on changing table to initiate game of Peekaboo*

■ *Laughs in response to getting tickled after diaper change is over*

SOCIAL-COMMUNICATION Beginning Skills

A 1   Turns and looks toward person speaking

A 2   Produces speech sounds

A 2.1 Coos and gurgles

A 3   Engages in vocal exchanges

A 3.1 Vocalizes to another person expressing positive affective state

A 3.2 Vocalizes to another person expressing negative affective state

A 4   Uses intentional gestures, vocalizations, and objects to communicate

A 4.4 Expresses negation or protests

B 1   Follows gaze to establish joint attention

B 1.1 Follows pointing gestures with eyes

B 1.2 Looks toward object

C 1.3 Uses consistent approximations for words or signs

C 1.4 Uses consistent consonant-vowel combinations

Embedded Learning Opportunities

■ *Looks at adult talking during diapering routine*

■ *Coos or babbles in response to adult's talking or singing while washing hands*

■ *Cries when time to leave toys for diaper change*

■ *Looks toward overhead mobile as adult looks at and points to it*

■ *Signs ALL DONE when diaper change is over*

COGNITIVE Beginning Skills

A 1   Orients to events or stimulation

A 1.1   Reacts to events or stimulation

B 1.1   Imitates novel simple motor action not already in repertoire

B 1.2   Imitates familiar simple motor action

B 2.1   Imitates novel vocalizations

B 2.2   Imitates familiar vocalizations

Embedded Learning Opportunities

■ *Moves toward diaper changing area when adult says "It's time for a diaper!"*

■ *Waves hand in front of nose and says "Phew!" after adult models it*

MATH Beginning Skills

A 1.2   Recites numbers 1–3

Embedded Learning Opportunities

■ *Says "1, 2, 3" before adult lifts them up to changing table*

TIER 1

■ UNIVERSAL STRATEGIES

These are best practices for ALL young children, with attention to meeting learning outcomes within daily routines and activities of family life and early childhood classrooms while promoting positive adult–child relationships and peer interactions.

Diapering, toileting, and handwashing are routines that happen frequently with infants and young toddlers. Diaper change time can be used as an opportunity for one-to-one teaching and provides valuable opportunities for social-emotional development. It is also a time to talk with the child and make eye contact to encourage language and vocabulary development. Following are some general suggestions:

▲ Label the necessary items for diaper changes (diapers, wipes, pants, socks) to help children develop vocabulary.

▲ Always carry out diaper changes consistently, telling children what is about to happen next, because this empowers them:

    △ Always tell children it is time for a diaper change before removing them from their current activity.

    △ Maintain the same routine each time, so children can predict what is coming next and start to participate in the steps.

▲ Make handwashing a part of all diapering and toileting routines:

    △ For children younger than 6 months, it is recommended that adults wash their own and infants' hands with a wipe or towel (e.g., Harms, Cryer, & Clifford, 2006).

    △ Children older than 6 months should wash their own hands with soap and running water after diaper changes, before and after eating, and when coming inside from outdoor play.

Interactions

The success of this routine depends strongly on adults' support and consistency throughout all parts. Following are some suggestions for interactions at the Beginning level:

▲ Use consistent vocabulary with children when discussing diaper changes, toileting, and handwashing.

▲ Use parallel talk to expand on children's vocabulary:

  △ Describe what you are doing ("I'm changing your diaper") or what the child is doing ("You're washing your hands").

  △ Sing songs to the child ("Wash, Wash, Wash Your Hands," sung to the tune of "Row, Row, Row Your Boat").

  △ Carry on a conversation, and wait for the child to respond through words, gestures, signs, or word approximations.

▲ Teach children expectations for the routine (they need to lie down while you are changing their diaper).

▲ Model the steps for handwashing to give children a visual to help them learn the routine.

▲ Incorporate mathematics into this routine by counting whenever possible (count the number of seconds children wash their hands or the number of toys on a mobile above a changing table).

▲ Give children immediate, consistent feedback about the routine they are learning ("I like the way you're washing your hands in the sink").

▲ Follow children's lead (if they say they need to wash their hands by holding up their dirty hands to show you, or if they say they need to use the bathroom, encourage them to use single words or signs for requests).

Environment and Materials

Toileting and handwashing should take place indoors in a bathroom at home, at child care, and during community outings. Diapering should take place on a changing table that meets safety regulations and that typically has a changing pad that can be washed and disinfected. Materials needed for this routine include soap, water, diapers, baby wipes, diaper ointment, diaper changing paper, and disinfectant. Following are some suggestions for environment and materials at the Beginning level:

▲ Mount a mobile, wind chime, or kite over the diapering area for visual interest.

▲ Lay children on a soft changing pad when changing diapers. Refrain from giving infants toys to play with during diapering, as it is an unsanitary practice.

▲ Use a poster showing proper handwashing procedures to help children learn the routine, or use posters with related nursery rhymes or songs (recite or sing the rhymes or songs to children during the routine).

■ FOCUSED STRATEGIES

These strategies are for teaching SOME children who are struggling with a component of a skill or whose development is stalled and who need extra help to catch up or keep up. The strategies include a variety of minor adaptations or modifications to daily routines, activities, and environments to meet targeted outcomes at home and in classrooms.

▲ Keep diapering predictable and consistent by following the same routine each time, using the same language, and using verbal cues to prompt each step of the routine.

▲ Use a different method to carry out the routine if children are struggling (when diapering an older infant or young toddler, try letting them stand during diaper changes if that makes them feel more comfortable).

▲ Provide books or pictures that show the steps of diapering, toileting, or washing hands, and talk about the steps.

▲ Use hand-over-hand to help children older than 6 months wash their hands.

▲ Use verbal prompts to remind children what they need to do to complete the routine ("Throw the paper towel in the garbage can").

▲ Let children who have difficulties transitioning from playing with a toy to diapering, toileting, or handwashing place the toy nearby and out of reach of other children while completing the routine.

▲ Play calming music or sounds during diaper changes to encourage calm and provide a soothing distraction.

▲ Teach children who cannot speak to use simple signs (MORE, ALL DONE) so they can communicate their preferences.

▲ Learn to recognize children's cues and preferences.

▲ Pair sign language with spoken words for children who are nonverbal or who have hearing impairments.

■ SPECIALIZED STRATEGIES

These strategies for teaching the FEW children who need intensive supports include a variety of specialized, individualized, precise evidence-based strategies to meet children's unique goals/outcomes:

▲ Let children touch or hold each item used in the diaper routine before it is used:

△ Allow the child to feel the wipe before wiping.

△ Let the child hold the new diaper before putting it on them.

▲ Use touch cues with verbal cues to let children who have visual impairments know what is happening during the routine:

△ Touch the child's bottom before removing their diaper while saying "Let's take off this wet [dirty] diaper."

△ Touch the child's hand before using a wipe and say "Now we'll wash your hands."

▲ Use graduated guidance to provide physical prompting for steps of handwashing that children cannot perform:

△ Say "Turn on the water," and give the child an opportunity to turn it on.

△ If the child doesn't turn on the water, point to the faucet and wait a short time for the child to turn it on.

△ If the child does not turn on the water, help them by placing your hands over theirs to turn it on.

AEPS-3 Curriculum Resources (Appendix A)

Appendix A in this volume contains numerous additional resources to supplement the AEPS-3 Curriculum. The first part of the appendix presents a list of general curriculum resources, and the second part provides lists of supplementary resources for each individual routine and activity.

AEPS-3 Skills Matrix (Appendix B)

The AEPS-3 Skills Matrix in Appendix B of this volume spotlights individual skills by showing functional application across all routines and activities. Each skills matrix (there are eight total, one for each of the test's eight developmental areas) allows you to select individual AEPS-3 items for children who require an intensive focus on a few skills across routines and activities. For children who have difficulty learning new skills at the level of individual AEPS-3 items, the Foundation Steps (FS) provide an even more granular breakdown of component subskills that are either a sequence of developmental precursors or steps in task analyses.

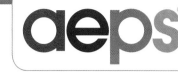

13

Dramatic Play

In Dramatic Play, children and others act out character parts (store clerk, farmer, doctor) by using imitation and imagination, often dressing up in clothes to act out roles. This type of play is often child led and can occur several times a day in any familiar setting. The activity changes over time as children's communication, cognitive, motor, and adaptive skills increase. The AEPS-3 Beginning level of Dramatic Play uses skills from eight developmental areas.

Concurrent Skills

The following concurrent skills are AEPS-3 skills that can be easily embedded and taught during regular occurrences of Dramatic Play.

FINE MOTOR Beginning Skills

A 1.1 Brings hands together near midline

A 2.1 Grasps hand-size object

A 2.2 Grasps small cylindrical object

A 2.3 Grasps pea-size object using fingers in raking or scratching movement

A 2.4 Grasps hand-size object using whole hand

A 3 Stacks objects

A 3.1 Releases object into targeted space

A 3.2 Releases object into nondefined space

B 1 Activates object with finger

B 1.1 Uses finger to point or touch

B 1.2 Uses hand to activate object

B 1.3 Uses fingers to explore object

B 2.1 Turns object using either hand

B 3.4 Holds object with one hand and manipulates object or produces action with other hand

B 3.5 Transfers object from hand to hand

Embedded Learning Opportunities

- *Holds toy phone or camera at midline*
- *Shakes hand-size musical instrument to make noise*
- *Grasps small cylindrical object (toy tool, toy doctor kit item, microphone)*
- *Stacks hats on dramatic play shelf*
- *Stacks dishes in dramatic play area*
- *Releases dishes into dish basket*
- *Uses finger to explore and activate toy cell phone*
- *Transfers toy camera from one hand to the other*

GROSS MOTOR Beginning Skills

A 4.4 Sits balanced without support

A 4.5 Sits balanced using hands for support

A 4.6 Holds head in midline when sitting supported

A 5 Gets out of chair

A 5.1 Sits down in chair

A 5.2 Maintains sitting position in chair

B 2 Stoops and regains balanced standing position

B 2.1 Rises from sitting to standing position

B 2.2 Stands unsupported

B 2.3 Pulls to standing position

B 2.4 Pulls to kneeling position

B 3.1 Walks without support

B 3.2 Walks with one-hand support

B 3.3 Walks with two-hand support

C 3.3 Pushes riding toy with feet while steering

C 3.4 Sits on riding toy or wagon while in motion

Embedded Learning Opportunities

- *Sits without support to play with baby doll*
- *Sits down on child-size chair beside table in dramatic play area and pretends to eat*
- *Bends down to get dropped toy*
- *Walks while pushing child-size shopping cart in dramatic play area*
- *Propels toy car with feet while steering*
- *Sits on riding toy while adult pushes it*

ADAPTIVE Beginning Skills

C 1.5 Takes off shoes

C 1.6 Takes off socks

C 1.7 Takes off hat

Embedded Learning Opportunities

- *Takes off hat when finished playing with it in dramatic play area*
- *Takes off shoes and socks to try on slippers in dramatic play area*

SOCIAL-EMOTIONAL Beginning Skills

A 2.2 Repeats part of interactive game or action in order to continue game or action

A 2.3 Responds to familiar game or action

C 1.3 Plays near one or two peers

D 3.3 Entertains self by playing with toys

D 4.2 Claims and defends possessions

Embedded Learning Opportunities

- *Gives adult phone to initiate pretend phone calls*
- *Says "Hi" and grabs phone when adult begins playing with phones*
- *Plays beside one or two friends in dramatic play area*
- *Plays alone in toy kitchen area*
- *Grabs toy from sibling who took it away and says "Mine!"*

SOCIAL-COMMUNICATION Beginning Skills

A 1 Turns and looks toward person speaking

A 2 Produces speech sounds

A 3 Engages in vocal exchanges

A 3.1 Vocalizes to another person expressing positive affective state

A 3.2 Vocalizes to another person expressing negative affective state

A 4 Uses intentional gestures, vocalizations, and objects to communicate

A 4.1 Makes requests of others

A 4.2 Makes choices to express preferences

A 4.3 Expresses desire to continue activity

A 4.4 Expresses negation or protests

B 1 Follows gaze to establish joint attention

B 1.1 Follows pointing gestures with eyes

B 1.2 Looks toward object

B 2.1 Recognizes own and familiar names

B 2.2 Responds to single-word directive

C 1.3 Uses consistent approximations for words or signs

C 1.4 Uses consistent consonant–vowel combinations

Embedded Learning Opportunities

- *Looks toward peer who is talking*
- *Laughs and coos when adult tries on hats*
- *Cries so adult will help take off costume*
- *Asks for doll by saying "Baby"*
- *Signs ALL DONE when ready to leave dramatic play area*
- *Looks toward and examines play clothes after adult says "Let's play with play clothes"*
- *Says "Mama" while pretending to talk to mom on phone*

COGNITIVE Beginning Skills

A 1 Orients to events or stimulation

A 1.1 Reacts to events or stimulation

A 2 Combines simple actions to examine people, animals, and objects

A 2.1 Uses sensory means to explore people, animals, and objects

B 1.1 Imitates novel simple motor action not already in repertoire

B 1.2 Imitates familiar simple motor action

B 2.1 Imitates novel vocalizations

B 2.2 Imitates familiar vocalizations

C 1.2 Locates hidden object

D 1 Uses object to obtain another object

D 1.1 Uses part of object or support to obtain another object

D 1.2 Retains one object when second object is obtained

D 2 Coordinates actions with objects to achieve new outcomes

D 2.1 Tries different simple actions to achieve goal

D 2.2 Uses simple actions on objects

E 1.2 Uses senses to explore

E 2.3 Makes observations

Embedded Learning Opportunities

- *Turns head and visually follows peer moving around in room*
- *Looks at adult using toy phone*
- *Opens and closes bags during dramatic play*
- *Signs MORE after adult taps fingertips together and says "more"*
- *Repeats "on" after adult says "Turn the camera on"*
- *Locates doctor kit after adult puts it back on shelf out of sight*
- *Uses spoon to get plate or pan from back of toy kitchen cabinet*
- *Uses sensory tube to knock out-of-reach items off dramatic play shelf*
- *Holds child-size cup in one hand and gets child-size plate for other hand*
- *Mouths pretend food*

LITERACY Beginning Skills

A 1.1 Participates in shared one-on-one reading

Embedded Learning Opportunities

■ *Sits in adult's lap while in dramatic play area to listen to book about community helpers*

MATH Beginning Skills

A 1.2 Recites numbers 1–3

Embedded Learning Opportunities

■ *Sings number song to "baby" in dramatic play area*

TIER 1

■ UNIVERSAL STRATEGIES

These are best practices for ALL young children, with attention to meeting learning outcomes within daily routines and activities of family life and early childhood classrooms while promoting positive adult–child relationships and peer interactions.

Dramatic play for infants and children at the Beginning level is child led but may require adults or peers to help or play with the child at times. Children at this level are becoming more mobile and able to engage in pretend play alone and with others. As their motor skills increase, they can sit, stand independently, walk, and steer a riding toy while pushing it with their feet. They are capable of picking up objects, manipulating objects using both hands, and transferring objects from hand to hand. Cognitively, children can imitate novel motor actions, words, and vocalizations. Their developing communication skills enable them to make requests of others and express their preferences. Socially, children gain the ability to play near peers, entertain themselves with toys, and claim or defend their possessions. Depending on the type of dramatic play, children may use their increased literacy and math skills too.

Interactions

Adults can support dramatic play in numerous ways. Following are some suggestions for interactions at the Beginning level:

▲ Follow children's lead and let them explore their environment.

▲ Place dramatic play items low enough in the play area that children are aware they can play with them.

▲ Introduce children to new items you bring out for them to play with, and teach expectations around how the items should be used and treated ("When you are finished playing with the puppets, put them away").

▲ Use a calm voice when speaking with children, and give them immediate, specific feedback ("You put the puppets away. Good job! Now you can play with something else").

▲ Model how to use new items while using parallel talk to explain what you are doing and what the item can be used for.

▲ Give children multiple opportunities throughout the day to engage in dramatic play.

▲ Make sure children are safe, and look for any teachable moments.

▲ Let older peers serve as role models for younger children during dramatic play.

Environment and Materials

At the Beginning level, dramatic play can occur both indoors and outdoors, in environments including home, child care, school, parks, and playgrounds. Possible materials for this routine are endless. Following are some suggestions for environment and routines at this level:

▲ Choose items for dramatic play with care:

   △ Keep children's ages, interests, and safety in mind (this is the age when children explore materials with their mouths).

   △ Provide appropriate materials for infants, such as dolls, soft animals, toy telephones, and toy pots and pans.

   △ Provide appropriate materials for toddlers, such as dress-up clothing, child-size play furniture, play foods, toy dishes and eating utensils, and a small playhouse.

▲ Consider a variety of sources for dramatic play items:

   △ New items purchased specifically for dramatic play

   △ Old items from around the house

   △ Inexpensive items from garage sales and thrift stores

   △ Pretend items fashioned from cardboard, wood, or PVC pipe

▲ Use your imagination when finding items for dramatic play, and consider children's interests.

▲ Create a themed dramatic play area (set up a pretend house with child-size kitchen, washer, dryer, dolls, toy food).

■ FOCUSED STRATEGIES

These strategies are for teaching SOME children who are struggling with a component of a skill or whose development is stalled and who need extra help to catch up or keep up. The strategies include a variety of minor adaptations or modifications to daily routines, activities, and environments to meet targeted outcomes at home and in classrooms.

▲ Offer multiple opportunities throughout the day to engage in dramatic play.

▲ Keep dramatic play area set up in your environment for a minimum of a week before changing it, because repetition is important.

▲ Provide multiples of favored dramatic play toys to help keep children from taking toys away from one another (give each child a baby doll to pretend to feed).

▲ Vary the materials used with children.

▲ Give children time to explore new items before becoming involved (some children may take a while to warm up to new materials or games and may require many opportunities to watch and observe before they participate):

   △ Model how to use materials, if necessary, to help a child become interested.

   △ Remove toys that children do not show interest in after a few days, and replace with other dramatic play toys.

▲ Pay close attention for times when babies are comfortable, alert, and ready to learn or play.

▲ Use a verbal prompt and a real object associated with the activity (toy telephone) to let children know it is time to transition from one activity to another.

▲ Teach children who cannot speak to use gestures or sign language so they can communicate their likes and dislikes.

▲ Use sign language for children who have hearing impairments, and explicitly model how to use items.

▲ Learn to recognize children's cues and preferences.

■ **SPECIALIZED STRATEGIES**

These strategies for teaching the FEW children who need intensive supports include a variety of specialized, individualized, precise evidence-based strategies to meet children's unique goals/outcomes:

▲ Make sure the dramatic play area is accessible for all children:

  △ Bring children who are not mobile to the dramatic play area, and give them toys to explore.

  △ Describe materials in detail for children who have visual impairments, and let them hold them.

  △ Make sure materials are within reach for children who have visual impairments and that the materials have auditory, tactile, or metallic properties (stuffed toys with bells inside them).

▲ Use environmental strategies to create opportunities for children to initiate expressive communication (withhold an object until the child gestures, signs, vocalizes, or reaches for it).

▲ Transport items used to help ease transitions (pacifier, chewie, blanket) from one environment to another.

AEPS-3 Curriculum Resources (Appendix A)

Appendix A in this volume contains numerous additional resources to supplement the AEPS-3 Curriculum. The first part of the appendix presents a list of general curriculum resources, and the second part provides lists of supplementary resources for each individual routine and activity.

AEPS-3 Skills Matrix (Appendix B)

The AEPS-3 Skills Matrix in Appendix B of this volume spotlights individual skills by showing functional application across all routines and activities. Each skills matrix (there are eight total, one for each of the test's eight developmental areas) allows you to select individual AEPS-3 items for children who require an intensive focus on a few skills across routines and activities. For children who have difficulty learning new skills at the level of individual AEPS-3 items, the Foundation Steps (*FS*) provide an even more granular breakdown of component subskills that are either a sequence of developmental precursors or steps in task analyses.

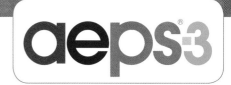

14

Dressing

The Dressing routine (which also includes undressing) changes significantly over time as infants begin to take greater interest in removing and putting on clothing as their fine motor, gross motor, adaptive, and cognitive abilities increase. Dressing involves important developmental skills that lead to much greater independence. This routine often occurs several times a day for young children, as when their soiled clothes need changing or they need more appropriate clothing as the schedule dictates (outdoors, bedtime, after bath, visiting friends, attending community activities). The AEPS-3 Beginning level of Dressing uses skills from seven developmental areas.

Concurrent Skills

The following concurrent skills are AEPS-3 skills that can be easily embedded and taught during regular occurrences of Dressing.

FINE MOTOR Beginning Skills

A 1 Makes directed batting or swiping movements with each hand

A 1.1 Brings hands together near midline

A 1.2 Makes directed movements with arms

A 2 Grasps pea-sized object

A 2.1 Grasps hand-size object

A 2.2 Grasps small cylindrical object

A 3.1 Releases object into targeted space

A 3.2 Releases object into nondefined space

B 1.1 Uses finger to point or touch

B 1.3 Uses fingers to explore object

B 2.1 Turns object using either hand

B 3.4 Holds object with one hand and manipulates object or produces action with other hand

B 3.5 Transfers object from hand to hand

Embedded Learning Opportunities

- *Bats at mobile above changing or dressing table*
- *Grasps knit hat with thumb and forefinger to pull it off*
- *Places socks in sock drawer*
- *Drops rattle on floor*
- *Explores clothing textures with fingers*
- *Transfers toy from one hand to other while getting dressed*

GROSS MOTOR Beginning Skills

A 1   Turns head, moves arms, and kicks legs
       independently of each other

A 1.1 Kicks legs

A 1.2 Waves arms

A 1.3 Turns head side to side

A 3   Rolls from back to stomach

A 3.2 Rolls from back or stomach to side

A 4   Assumes balanced sitting position

A 4.4 Sits balanced without support

A 4.5 Sits balanced using hands for support

A 4.6 Holds head in midline when sitting supported

A 5   Gets out of chair

A 5.1 Sits down in chair

A 5.2 Maintains sitting position in chair

B 2   Stoops and regains balanced standing position

B 2.1 Rises from sitting to standing position

B 2.2 Stands unsupported

B 2.3 Pulls to standing position

B 3.1 Walks without support

B 3.2 Walks with one-hand support

B 3.3 Walks with two-hand support

Embedded Learning Opportunities

- *Turns head and kicks legs when adult is talking*
- *Rolls from back to stomach on floor while adult tries to dress child*
- *Sits down in child-size chair so adult can put on their shoes*
- *Sits balanced with or without support while getting dressed*
- *Pulls to standing on dresser*
- *Walks around helping adult get clothes out of drawers*

ADAPTIVE Beginning Skills

C 1.5 Takes off shoes

C 1.6 Takes off socks

C 1.7 Takes off hat

Embedded Learning Opportunities

- *Takes off shoes, socks, hat to help adult with undressing*

SOCIAL-EMOTIONAL Beginning Skills

A 1   Initiates positive social behavior toward familiar adult

A 1.1 Responds appropriately to familiar adult's affective tone

A 1.2 Responds to familiar adult's positive social behavior

A 2   Maintains social interaction with familiar adult

A 2.1 Initiates simple social interaction with familiar adult

A 2.2 Repeats part of interactive game or action in order to continue game or action

A 2.3 Responds to familiar game or action

B 2.2 Seeks comfort, closeness, or physical contact from familiar adult

B 2.3 Responds appropriately to soothing by adult

Embedded Learning Opportunities

- *Gives adult hug and kiss*
- *Babbles back and forth with adult*
- *Claps hands to continue playing Pat-a-cake*
- *Crawls or walks to bedroom when adult says "It's time to get dressed"*
- *Grabs blanket and sits in adult's lap after dressing*

SOCIAL-COMMUNICATION Beginning Skills

A 1	Turns and looks toward person speaking
A 1.1	Quiets to familiar voice
A 2	Produces speech sounds
A 2.1	Coos and gurgles
A 3	Engages in vocal exchanges
A 3.1	Vocalizes to another person expressing positive affective state
A 3.2	Vocalizes to another person expressing negative affective state
A 4	Uses intentional gestures, vocalizations, and objects to communicate
A 4.1	Makes requests of others
A 4.2	Makes choices to express preferences
A 4.4	Expresses negation or protests
B 1	Follows gaze to establish joint attention
B 1.1	Follows pointing gestures with eyes
B 1.2	Looks toward object
B 2.1	Recognizes own and familiar names
B 2.2	Responds to single-word directive
C 1.3	Uses consistent approximations for words or signs
C 1.4	Uses consistent consonant–vowel combinations

Embedded Learning Opportunities

- *Looks at adult while adult sings songs*
- *Coos, listens as adult imitates child, and responds by cooing again*
- *Cries when adult gets child dressed and undressed*
- *Signs MORE to ask adult to keep putting on lotion*
- *Looks at object when adult says "Go get that, please"*
- *Sits down when adult says "Sit, please"*
- *Says "Mama" when mother walks into room*
- *Says "Go bye-bye" when adult begins putting on coat*

COGNITIVE Beginning Skills

A 1	Orients to events or stimulation
A 1.1	Reacts to events or stimulation
A 2.1	Uses sensory means to explore people, animals, and objects
B 1.1	Imitates novel simple motor action not already in repertoire
B 1.2	Imitates familiar simple motor action
B 2.1	Imitates novel vocalizations
B 2.2	Imitates familiar vocalizations
C 1.2	Locates hidden object
D 1	Uses object to obtain another object
D 1.1	Uses part of object or support to obtain another object
D 1.2	Retains one object when second object is obtained
D 2	Coordinates actions with objects to achieve new outcomes
D 2.1	Tries different simple actions to achieve goal
D 2.2	Uses simple actions on objects
E 1.2	Uses senses to explore

Embedded Learning Opportunities

- *Reaches for adult's face as adult dresses child*
- *Looks and bats at mobile above changing table*
- *Puts socks on head after adult does so jokingly*
- *Says "bababa," listens as adult imitates babbling, and babbles "bababa" again*
- *Finds clothing item adult hides under blanket*
- *Uses one shoe to pull second shoe closer*
- *Holds one shoe while picking up sock with other hand*
- *Puts shoe on top of foot, then foot on top of shoe, when trying to put shoe on*
- *Uses senses to explore different clothing textures*

MATH Beginning Skills

A 1.2 Recites numbers 1–3

Embedded Learning Opportunities

■ *Recites numbers with adult while getting dressed*

TIER 1

■ UNIVERSAL STRATEGIES

These are best practices for ALL young children, with attention to meeting learning outcomes within daily routines and activities of family life and early childhood classrooms while promoting positive adult–child relationships and peer interactions.

Participation at the Beginning level involves more undressing or taking off clothing than dressing. As fine motor skills develop, young children become able to achieve motor positions that let them participate more actively, engage and interact with adults, and react to and imitate actions that support an increase in their dressing and undressing skills.

For young children, dressing occurs many times daily, as infants' outfits typically are changed at least once a day, and clothes are removed and replaced during diapering and bathing. Dressing in the very earliest stages of development is a daily experience carried out primarily by parents and other adults. Young children quickly use their developing motor and cognitive skills (reaching, grasping, sitting, standing, attending, imitating) to participate in dressing. In addition to building a foundation for independent self-care, dressing provides valuable opportunities for very young children to practice important social and communication skills.

Dressing is a movement-oriented routine with fairly energetic activities that can be fun and pleasurable but that can also cause stress or upset. Keeping routines consistent with an emphasis on positive interactions allows children to anticipate an enjoyable experience while learning new ways to move their bodies to dress and undress. Ideally, dressing provides a context for enjoyable face-to-face interactions rather than being an activity to be completed before the fun begins.

Interactions

Taking the time to emphasize human interactions during this routine, rather than focusing on getting through the process of dressing and undressing, is an important way adults can support self-regulation and teach children how to calm down during times of upset. Dressing thus becomes a time for children to learn much more than putting on and taking off clothing. Following are some suggested interactions for the Beginning level of this routine:

▲ Use a calm, soothing voice to describe in simple language what is going on during dressing and undressing, and keep the focus on interactions.

▲ Pace the experience to avoid startling infants and to give them time to react and adjust to what is happening:

△ Take it slow, and pay attention to whether the child is getting stressed or uncomfortable.

△ Pause between pulling a shirt over the child's head and pushing their arms through the sleeves to make eye contact, smile, and say, "There you are, I see you!"

▲ Play simple social games while dressing to provide a fun distraction from movements that might be unfamiliar or uncomfortable for children (play Peekaboo while putting on a shirt, tickle an infant's stomach before pulling their shirt down).

▲ Talk about and describe different parts of the routine to help children notice the colors and textures of their clothes, learn labels for movements ("Push," "Arms up"), and build early vocabulary.

Environment and Materials

Parents and other adults can set the stage for successful dressing by using timing, simple materials, and a positive tone to maximize the child's comfort level and provide a relaxed start for the routine. Following are some suggestions for environment and materials for the Beginning level:

▲ Keep the room at a comfortable temperature.

▲ Start the process with an enthusiastic "Let's get you dressed!"

▲ Allow plenty of time for the routine.

▲ Avoid trying to dress a child who is already upset.

▲ Allow a few minutes after an infant wakes up before starting to dress them.

▲ Provide a clean, soft surface for the changing table or a floor covering that feels nice against sensitive skin, especially for children who are not yet sitting.

▲ Arrange all wipes, creams, and clean clothes nearby before starting to undress infants for diaper changes. This allows the adult to focus on child safety and social interactions rather than on locating clothing with one hand while managing a bare, squirming infant with the other and helps the routine go much more smoothly and quickly.

■ FOCUSED STRATEGIES

These strategies are for teaching SOME children who are struggling with a component of a skill or whose development is stalled and who need extra help to catch up or keep up. The strategies include a variety of minor adaptations or modifications to daily routines, activities, and environments to meet targeted outcomes at home and in classrooms.

▲ Accommodate young children's textile sensitivities by buying clothing in preferred fabrics or styles (soft fleece pants, shirts without buttons).

▲ Make sure the environment meets children's specific needs:

△ Keep the room at a comfortable temperature (not too cold).

△ Make sure changing tables, if used, have a soft, comfortable surface.

△ Try dressing the child on the floor or a low bed if they do not like being up high on a changing table and feel safer lower down.

△ Create a dynamic, interesting space for dressing:

▷ Hang posters for children to look at.

▷ Try hanging streamers, balloons, mobiles, or windsocks from the ceiling, because their movement is engaging and encourages children to reach and grasp.

▲ Take breaks while dressing and undressing if children seem overwhelmed:

△ Hold and soothe the child for a moment.

△ Start playing a game as soon as the child begins to become upset to help prevent full-blown distress.

▲ Let children who can sit or stand remain upright during dressing rather than having them lie on their back for the entire routine.

▲ Allow extra time for dressing and undressing when prompting children for new responses.

▲ Keep dressing predictable and consistent by following the same routine each day and using verbal cues to prompt each step.

▲ Use consistent word labels for articles of clothing and prompting.

▲ Limit choices so as not to overwhelm children (give two options to let them show their preference in clothing).

▲ Focus on social and communication skills during the routine:

△ Use dressing as a time to engage the child's attention with vocal play.

△ Play simple games like Peekaboo.

▲ Teach children who cannot speak to use simple signs (MORE, ALL DONE) so they can communicate their preferences.

▲ Learn to recognize children's cues and preferences.

▲ Pair sign language with spoken words for children who are nonverbal or who have hearing impairments.

■ SPECIALIZED STRATEGIES

These strategies for teaching the FEW children who need intensive supports include a variety of specialized, individualized, precise evidence-based strategies to meet children's unique goals/outcomes.

▲ Plan extra time for dressing and undressing.

▲ Let very young children focus on only one piece of clothing while dressing (dress the child efficiently except for one clothing item, such as socks or shirt, and let the child focus on just that one item).

▲ Position children for maximum stability during dressing and undressing (with the child lying down or sitting on the floor with their back against the wall).

▲ Combine simple verbal cues with prompts at each step in the routine (say "Lift up your legs" while lifting the child's legs to change a diaper or "Push your arm through" while pulling the child's arm into a sleeve).

▲ Use the routine as a context for teaching foundational skills such as sitting, standing, grasping, responding to adult interactions, and imitating sounds and motor actions.

▲ Give children plenty of time before dressing and after verbal prompts so they can process what is going to happen ("We're about to put on our clothes now").

▲ Sing the same song every time to signal the transition to dressing.

▲ For children who have sensory impairments, combine simple verbal cues with touch cues at each step in the routine (touch baby's bottom and say "Lift up your legs" while lifting the child's legs to change a diaper, or touch baby's forearm and say "Push your arm through" while pulling the child's arm into a sleeve).

▲ For children who have vision impairments:

△ Explain the routine in detail, and let the child hold the materials being used.

△ Assist from behind using hand-under-hand so the child can feel the task's natural movements.

▲ For children who are nonverbal or who have hearing impairments:

△ Use sign language, and show the child each item before putting it on.

▲ For children who have muscular disorders:

△ Position the child comfortably for dressing (on a soft bed).

△ Use massage to help loosen tight muscles.

AEPS-3 Curriculum Resources (Appendix A)

Appendix A in this volume contains numerous additional resources to supplement the AEPS-3 Curriculum. The first part of the appendix presents a list of general curriculum resources, and the second part provides lists of supplementary resources for each individual routine and activity.

AEPS-3 Skills Matrix (Appendix B)

The AEPS-3 Skills Matrix in Appendix B of this volume spotlights individual skills by showing functional application across all routines and activities. Each skills matrix (there are eight total, one for each of the test's eight developmental areas) allows you to select individual AEPS-3 items for children who require an intensive focus on a few skills across routines and activities. For children who have difficulty learning new skills at the level of individual AEPS-3 items, the Foundation Steps (*FS*) provide an even more granular breakdown of component subskills that are either a sequence of developmental precursors or steps in task analyses.

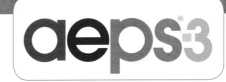

15

Field Trips

The Field Trips activity offers opportunities for children and adults to explore and learn about their community and society together. During field trips and outings, children discover new experiences and environments they may not have access to in their usual daily routines. At the Beginning level, this activity may involve stroller rides, walking, biking, or motor transport with adults. It may mean going to a library, park, playground, recreational area, or museum. Depending on the adult and child, a field trip may take place several times a week. Types of outings taken evolve over time as children become more aware of their environment and develop cognitive, social-communication, and social-emotional skills that allow them to participate more actively in the activity. The AEPS-3 Beginning level of this routine uses skills from eight developmental areas.

Concurrent Skills

The following concurrent skills are AEPS-3 skills that can be easily embedded and taught during regular occurrences of Field Trips.

FINE MOTOR	Beginning Skills

A 1 Makes directed batting or swiping movements with each hand

A 1.1 Brings hands together near midline

A 1.2 Makes directed movements with arms

A 2 Grasps pea-size object

A 2.1 Grasps hand-size object

A 2.2 Grasps small cylindrical object

A 2.3 Grasps pea-size object using fingers in raking or scratching movement

A 2.4 Grasps hand-size object using whole hand

A 3 Stacks objects

A 3.1 Releases object into targeted space

A 3.2 Releases object into nondefined space

B 1 Activates object with finger

B 1.1 Uses finger to point or touch

B 1.2 Uses hand to activate object

B 1.3 Uses fingers to explore object

B 2.1 Turns object using either hand

B 3.4 Holds object with one hand and manipulates object or produces action with other hand

B 3.5 Transfers object from hand to hand

Embedded Learning Opportunities

- *Grasps rattle while in stroller*
- *Grasps Cheerio while having quick snack*
- *Replaces books on library shelf after storytime*
- *Pushes elevator button to get to top floor of museum or library*
- *Explores items of different textures (sand at playground, bubbles in museum's bubble room)*
- *Transfers comfort item (stuffed toy bunny) to other hand to hold adult's hand*

GROSS MOTOR Beginning Skills

A 1   Turns head, moves arms, and kicks legs independently of each other

A 1.1   Kicks legs

A 1.2   Waves arms

A 1.3   Turns head side to side

A 2   Puts weight on one hand or arm while reaching with opposite hand

A 2.1   Remains propped on extended arms with head lifted

A 2.2   Remains propped on nonextended forearms with head lifted

A 3   Rolls from back to stomach

A 3.1   Rolls from stomach to back

A 3.2   Rolls from back or stomach to side

A 4   Assumes balanced sitting position

A 4.1   Assumes hands-and-knees position from sitting

A 4.2   Regains balanced, upright sitting position after reaching across body

A 4.3   Regains balanced, upright sitting position after leaning left, right, and forward

A 4.4   Sits balanced without support

A 4.5   Sits balanced using hands for support

A 4.6   Holds head in midline when sitting supported

A 5   Gets out of chair

A 5.1   Sits down in chair

A 5.2   Maintains sitting position in chair

B 1   Creeps forward using alternating arm and leg movements

B 1.1   Rocks while in creeping position

B 1.2   Assumes creeping position

B 1.3   Crawls forward on stomach

B 1.4   Pivots on stomach

B 2   Stoops and regains balanced standing position

B 2.1   Rises from sitting to standing position

B 2.2   Stands unsupported

B 2.3   Pulls to standing position

B 3.1   Walks without support

B 3.2   Walks with one-hand support

B 3.3   Walks with two-hand support

B 3.4   Cruises

B 6.3   Jumps down with support

C 1.6   Throws or rolls ball at target with two hands

C 3.3   Pushes riding toy with feet while steering

C 3.4   Sits on riding toy or in wagon while in motion

Embedded Learning Opportunities

■ *Turns head while lying on picnic blanket at park and watching others play*

■ *Turns head to look at new environment (zoo, museum)*

■ *Rolls over to get bottle placed out of reach on picnic blanket*

■ *Sits to listen to adult read at library*

■ *Sits in wagon independently while being pulled to park*

■ *Bends to pick up item (toy, book, block) at library storytime*

■ *Walks around playground, museum, store*

■ *Cruises playground equipment while at park*

■ *Jumps off playground equipment with support*

■ *Pushes riding toy with feet around park*

ADAPTIVE Beginning Skills

A 1   Uses lips to take semisolid foods off eating utensil

A 1.1 Swallows semisolid foods

A 1.2 Swallows liquids

A 2.2 Eats crisp foods

A 2.3 Eats soft and dissolvable foods

A 3.2 Eats with fingers

A 3.3 Accepts food presented on eating utensils

A 4.1 Drinks from cup with spouted lid

A 4.2 Drinks from container held by adult

C 1.6 Takes off socks

C 1.7 Takes off hat

Embedded Learning Opportunities

■ *Eats bananas, peeled apple slices, cantaloupe while on outing with adult*

■ *Eats crackers, rice cakes, cookies while on outing with adult*

■ *Drinks water from spouted cup while on outing with adult*

■ *Takes off socks and hat upon returning home from family outing*

SOCIAL-EMOTIONAL Beginning Skills

A 1   Initiates positive social behavior toward familiar adult

A 1.1 Responds appropriately to familiar adult's affective tone

A 1.2 Responds to familiar adult's positive social behavior

A 2   Maintains social interaction with familiar adult

A 2.1 Initiates simple social interaction with familiar adult

A 2.2 Repeats part of interactive game or action in order to continue game or action

A 2.3 Responds to familiar game or action

B 2.2 Seeks comfort, closeness, or physical contact from familiar adult

B 2.3 Responds appropriately to soothing by adult

C 1.3 Plays near one or two peers

D 3.3 Entertains self by playing with toys

D 4.2 Claims and defends possessions

Embedded Learning Opportunities

■ *Plays Peekaboo with adult while at park*

■ *Calms when comforted by adult after falling down*

■ *Says "Go!" to make adult chase them*

■ *Calms when scared about being in new environment*

■ *Plays with peer on playground equipment*

■ *Says "Mine!" when another child tries to take their toy*

SOCIAL-COMMUNICATION Beginning Skills

A 1   Turns and looks toward person speaking

A 1.1   Quiets to familiar voice

A 2   Produces speech sounds

A 2.1   Coos and gurgles

A 3   Engages in vocal exchanges

A 3.1   Vocalizes to another person expressing positive affective state

A 3.2   Vocalizes to another person expressing negative affective state

A 4   Uses intentional gestures, vocalizations, and objects to communicate

A 4.1   Makes requests of others

A 4.2   Makes choices to express preferences

A 4.3   Expresses desire to continue activity

A 4.4   Expresses negation or protests

B 1   Follows gaze to establish joint attention

B 1.1   Follows pointing gestures with eyes

B 1.2   Looks toward object

B 2.1   Recognizes own and familiar names

B 2.2   Responds to single-word directive

C 1.3   Uses consistent approximations for words or signs

C 1.4   Uses consistent consonant-vowel combinations

Embedded Learning Opportunities

- *Looks at adult when adult calls their name*
- *Laughs when adult plays Peekaboo during picnic*
- *Cries to express distress when unable to get off playground equipment*
- *Signs MORE to continue getting pushed on swing*
- *Chooses to read books instead of play at library*
- *Looks at adult and points to swing*
- *Looks at slide after adult says "Let's go down the slide!"*
- *Says "ba" for ball whenever referring to ball*

COGNITIVE Beginning Skills

A 1   Orients to events or stimulation

A 1.1   Reacts to events or stimulation

A 2   Combines simple actions to examine people, animals, and objects

A 2.1   Uses sensory means to explore people, animals, and objects

B 1.1   Imitates novel simple motor action not already in repertoire

B 1.2   Imitates familiar simple motor action

B 2.1   Imitates novel vocalizations

B 2.2   Imitates familiar vocalizations

D 2   Coordinates actions with objects to achieve new outcomes

D 2.1   Tries different simple actions to achieve goal

D 2.2   Uses simple actions on objects

E 1.2   Uses senses to explore

E 2.3   Makes observations

Embedded Learning Opportunities

- *Comes to adult when adult calls their name*
- *Kicks legs upon seeing stroller and recognizing it means going outside*
- *Imitates adult by waving hello and goodbye*
- *Says "ball" after adult says "Look, a ball!"*
- *Kicks and throws ball at playground*
- *Points at bird and says "bird"*
- *Bends to feel wet grass on playground*

LITERACY Beginning Skills

A 1.1 Participates in shared one-on-one reading

Embedded Learning Opportunities

■ *Participates in reading experiences while at library*

MATH Beginning Skills

A 1.2 Recites numbers 1–3

Embedded Learning Opportunities

■ *Counts fish with adult at aquarium*

■ *Repeats "1, 2, 3, go!" before going down slide*

TIER 1

■ UNIVERSAL STRATEGIES

These are best practices for ALL young children, with attention to meeting learning outcomes within daily routines and activities of family life and early childhood classrooms while promoting positive adult–child relationships and peer interactions.

For young children at the Beginning level, field trips/community outings might include stroller rides, walks or drives to a park or playground, library activities such as storytime, visits to community points of interest such as museums or zoos, or errands with adults to the grocery store or bank. Young children start learning about community, society, and social norms by using their senses, motor skills, and social-communication skills to explore their surroundings. Adults can support early learning during field trips in many ways (detailed further in later sections), such as by following the child's lead, using parallel talk, modeling actions and behavior, asking questions, scaffolding responses, and attending to children's prior learning.

Interactions

Familiar adults may have the most success introducing infants and young children to new places and experiences. Following are some suggested interactions for the Beginning level:

▲ Embed opportunities to use a variety of developmental skills in each field trip:

  △ Use math talk to incorporate counting.

  △ Address children's feelings to help promote social-emotional development.

  △ Read books to encourage early literacy.

  △ Offer a wide range of experiences with a variety of materials to develop fine and gross motor skills.

▲ Make sure children are well fed, rested, and wearing comfortable clothes for new experiences so they will be active, alert, and ready.

▲ Give young children opportunities to observe older or more skilled peers to help them learn new skills without direct instruction.

▲ Give infants adequate time to experiment with and explore new surroundings and materials before attempting to teach or model new skills. Observing children's existing skills and knowledge enables adults to scaffold new learning.

▲ Inform children in advance of field trips about plans and expectations:

△ Where and when they will go

△ What it will be like when they get there

△ What the rules and expectations are for their behavior (use quiet voices in the library, stay close to adults, hold a hand when crossing the street).

Environment and Materials

Following are some suggestions for Beginning level environments and materials:

▲ Offer a variety of experiences and materials to encourage young children to explore and experiment with textures, sizes, and shapes while using their fine motor, gross motor, cognitive, and social-emotional skills.

▲ Stay with children during outings, and use parallel talk and scaffolded responses to help them understand what they are exploring.

▲ Visit different parks, playgrounds, and recreational areas to let children experience a variety of play surfaces (sand, wood chips, rubber chips, rocks).

▲ Plan ahead, and always take along emergency contact information in case it is needed.

■ FOCUSED STRATEGIES

These strategies are for teaching SOME children who are struggling with a component of a skill or whose development is stalled and who need extra help to catch up or keep up. The strategies include a variety of minor adaptations or modifications to daily routines, activities, and environments to meet targeted outcomes at home and in classrooms.

▲ Talk or sing to children to let them know where you are going.

▲ Alert children about upcoming transitions more than once if necessary.

▲ Take along friends or siblings who are more socially competent than younger children to decrease distractions during outings and model appropriate behavior.

▲ Take along materials children are comfortable using in their natural environment and incorporate ways to use them in the new environment to help children become comfortable there.

▲ Pay close attention for times when infants are comfortable, alert, and ready to learn or play.

▲ Allow children to become comfortable in new environments at their own pace. Some children may take a while to warm up to new environments, people, or materials and may need many opportunities to watch and observe before becoming involved.

▲ For children who are nonverbal or who have hearing impairments,

△ Teach simple signs (MORE, ALL DONE) so the child can communicate their preferences.

△ Learn to recognize the child's cues and preferences.

△ Pair sign language with spoken words.

■ SPECIALIZED STRATEGIES

These strategies for teaching the FEW children who need intensive supports include a variety of specialized, individualized, precise evidence-based strategies to meet children's unique goals/outcomes:

▲ Check ahead of time to make sure new environments are accessible to children who have motor, vision, hearing, or sensory needs, and make provisions as needed.

▲ For children who tend to become easily overwhelmed by sensory stimuli,

△ Locate quiet or less busy playgrounds, parks, and recreational areas to explore.

▲ For children who have vision impairments,

△ Explain in detail everything that is happening in the child's surroundings.

△ Let the child explore new environments at their own pace because new places may be overwhelming.

▲ For children who have mobility needs,

△ Provide adapted equipment for playgrounds if needed (adapted swing, raised sand table, ramped slide for children in wheelchairs).

▲ For children who need assistance with motor skills,

△ Use hand-over-hand guidance if needed (to turn pages in a board book in the library, to shovel sand on the playground, to take off shoes upon returning from an outing).

△ Fade hand-over-hand guidance using most-to-least prompting.

▲ Make sure the ratio of adults to children who may need extra assistance in new environments is one to one (children who have vision impairments who need extra support exploring the environment).

AEPS-3 Curriculum Resources (Appendix A)

Appendix A in this volume contains numerous additional resources to supplement the AEPS-3 Curriculum. The first part of the appendix presents a list of general curriculum resources, and the second part provides lists of supplementary resources for each individual routine and activity.

AEPS-3 Skills Matrix (Appendix B)

The AEPS-3 Skills Matrix in Appendix B of this volume spotlights individual skills by showing functional application across all routines and activities. Each skills matrix (there are eight total, one for each of the test's eight developmental areas) allows you to select individual AEPS-3 items for children who require an intensive focus on a few skills across routines and activities. For children who have difficulty learning new skills at the level of individual AEPS-3 items, the Foundation Steps (*FS*) provide an even more granular breakdown of component subskills that are either a sequence of developmental precursors or steps in task analyses.

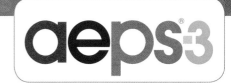

16

Math

Math is an important element in many children's daily routines. Acquiring early math skills is essential in building a strong foundation for school readiness. Math activities can be embedded in any routine, at any time, in any environment, multiple times a day. Peer and adult guidance and modeling may be needed to help children relate their daily experiences to math. This activity changes over time as children develop cognitive and social-communication skills. The AEPS-3 Beginning level of Math uses skills from six developmental areas.

Concurrent Skills

The following concurrent skills are AEPS-3 skills that can be easily embedded and taught during regular occurrences of Math. Many of the concurrent goals and objectives in this range are foundational skills for specific math concepts and later, math-related play goals.

FINE MOTOR Beginning Skills

A 2   Grasps pea-size object

A 2.1 Grasps hand-size object

A 2.2 Grasps small cylindrical object

A 2.3 Grasps pea-size object using fingers in raking or scratching movement

A 2.4 Grasps hand-size object using whole hand

A 3   Stacks objects

B 1   Activates object with finger

B 1.3 Uses fingers to explore object

B 2.1 Turns object using either hand

B 3.5 Transfers object from hand to hand

Embedded Learning Opportunities

- *Uses fingers and hands to manipulate and explore objects at sensory table*
- *Grasps block and transfers it to other hand before dropping it into bucket*
- *Activates mechanical toy with numbers on it by pushing buttons with one finger*

GROSS MOTOR Beginning Skills

A 5   Gets out of chair

A 5.1   Sits down in chair

A 5.2   Maintains sitting position in chair

B 2.2   Stands unsupported

C 1.6   Throws or rolls ball at target with two hands

Embedded Learning Opportunities

■ *Plays with manipulatives while standing at table or sitting on floor*

■ *Sits in highchair while adult counts out three crackers*

■ *Throws ball with numbers on it overhead into yard*

SOCIAL-EMOTIONAL Beginning Skills

A 2   Maintains social interaction with familiar adult

A 2.1   Initiates simple social interaction with familiar adult

A 2.2   Repeats part of interactive game or action in order to continue game or action

A 2.3   Responds to familiar game or action

C 1.3   Plays near one or two peers

D 3.3   Entertains self by playing with toys

D 4.2   Claims and defends possessions

Embedded Learning Opportunities

■ *Completes simple puzzle with help from adult*

■ *Sits on floor near peer as each plays with pop-up box*

■ *Says "Mine!" when another child attempts to take away toy*

SOCIAL-COMMUNICATION Beginning Skills

A 4   Uses intentional gestures, vocalizations, and objects to communicate

A 4.1   Makes requests of others

A 4.2   Makes choices to express preferences

B 1.1   Follows pointing gestures with eyes

B 1.2   Looks toward object

Embedded Learning Opportunities

■ *Makes eye contact and holds up shape to tell adult help is needed with shape sorter*

■ *Chooses between two types of manipulatives by pointing to one*

COGNITIVE Beginning Skills

A 1   Orients to events or stimulation

A 1.1   Reacts to events or stimulation

A 2   Combines simple actions to examine people, animals, and objects

A 2.1   Uses sensory means to explore people, animals, and objects

B 1.1   Imitates novel simple motor action not already in repertoire

B 1.2   Imitates familiar simple motor action

B 2.1   Imitates novel vocalizations

B 2.2   Imitates familiar vocalizations

E 2.3   Makes observations

Embedded Learning Opportunities

- *Watches nearby peer build tower and startles when it falls*
- *Helps adult build tower by adding blocks*
- *Picks up two hand-size balls of different textures, looks at them closely, and feels them*
- *Imitates adult by putting one block on top of another after adult does so*
- *Observes block tower falling and claps hands*

MATH Beginning Skills

A 1.2   Recites numbers 1–3

Embedded Learning Opportunities

- *Holds up arms and anticipates being picked up as adult counts, "1, 2, 3, up!"*

TIER 1

UNIVERSAL STRATEGIES

These are best practices for ALL young children, with attention to meeting learning outcomes within daily routines and activities of family life and early childhood classrooms while promoting positive adult–child relationships and peer interactions:

▲   Make sure children are active, alert, and ready to learn when introducing new materials and concepts.

▲   Provide adequate time for children to experiment with and explore new objects and materials on their own before attempting to teach or model new skills and before expecting children to initiate interactions.

▲   Incorporate a range of math experiences throughout the daily schedule rather than reserving math for a separate place and time.

▲   Use repetition to encourage recognition of quantity words and concepts, presenting songs, rhymes, words, activities, and materials multiple times and watching for signs of familiarity.

▲   Encourage children to observe other children playing with and exploring materials, and let very young children interact with slightly older or more skilled peers so they can observe and imitate new skills.

▲   Try using all environments and activities to help develop early math concepts.

Interactions

Infants and children at the Beginning level become acquainted with math most effectively through interactions with familiar adults. Following are some suggested interactions for this routine:

▲ Use math talk to embed math ideas and math learning in all areas of play and daily routines:

   △ Take advantage of opportunities to incorporate counting into the daily routine (count out crackers for a snack, count fingers when washing hands).

   △ Model quantitative language (say "All gone!" "No more!" and "More?" when an infant finishes their snack).

   △ Use math concepts when describing objects (big/little toy truck) to help build foundational skills for the very young.

   △ Sing nursery songs with numbers ("One, Two, Buckle My Shoe," "The Ants Go Marching").

   △ Count to three when picking children up ("1, 2, 3, up!").

▲ Read books with numbers to very young children so they have an opportunity to hear, see, and use number words.

Environment and Materials

Following are some suggestions for environment and materials at the Beginning level of this routine:

▲ Make sure the materials and concepts incorporated are of interest to very young children:

   △ Hand-size blocks in many shapes and sizes

   △ Recycled containers (sanitized and washed according to health and safety standards)

   △ Bath toys that are easy to clean

   △ Foam bath letters and numbers

   △ Mixing spoons with different handle lengths

   △ Child-size cups

   △ Teething toys

▲ Ensure that no item is a choking hazard.

▲ Incorporate math into playground activities (by counting before going down the slide or when filling and dumping buckets in the sand box).

▲ Develop early math concepts during free play by letting children count and stack blocks, read books that include numbers and counting, and play with ring tower, shape sorter, and simple puzzles.

▲ Incorporate sequencing and counting into diaper changes and dressing:

   △ Use sequencing words such as *first, next,* and *finally* throughout the process.

   △ Count snaps or buttons while fastening them.

■ FOCUSED STRATEGIES

These strategies are for teaching SOME children who are struggling with a component of a skill or whose development is stalled and who need extra help to catch up or keep up. The strategies include a variety of minor adaptations or modifications to daily routines, activities, and environments to meet targeted outcomes at home and in classrooms.

▲ Use repetition to encourage children to recognize quantity words and concepts:

△ Present songs, rhymes, words, activities, and materials multiple times, and watch for signs of familiarity.

△ Embed math-related opportunities in multiple daily routines so children get to hear, see, and engage with numbers, counting, and quantitative language many times each day.

▲ Vary the environments where math occurs, using settings where young children are sitting or standing, active, and alert, such as outdoors during playtime or in a highchair.

▲ Pay close attention for times when infants are comfortable, alert, and ready to learn or play, because some may take a while to warm up to new materials or games and need many opportunities to watch and observe before becoming involved.

▲ Start counting to 3 with rhymes and songs that use the child's fingers, toes, arms, and legs. Once the child seems to anticipate and engage with counting, expand to counting other people's fingers and toes or familiar objects such as finger foods and blocks.

▲ Teach children who cannot speak to use simple signs (MORE, ALL DONE) so they can communicate their preferences.

▲ Learn to recognize children's cues and preferences.

▲ Pair sign language with spoken words for children who are nonverbal or who have hearing impairments.

■ SPECIALIZED STRATEGIES

These strategies for teaching the FEW children who need intensive supports include a variety of specialized, individualized, precise evidence-based strategies to meet children's unique goals/outcomes:

▲ Accommodate the needs of children who have limited spans of attention and engagement by integrating counting into soothing activities (rocking, patting, or rubbing the child's back) instead of presenting quantity words and materials directly.

▲ Provide hand-over-hand assistance to help children clap in rhythm with music.

▲ Count children's steps ("1, 2, 3!") while teaching walking.

▲ Offer a structured choice for preferred snacks to begin building an understanding that 2 is more than 1:

△ Ask, "Do you want ONE cracker, or TWO crackers?"

△ Respond by offering whichever option the child chose and naming the choice ("Here's ONE cracker").

▲ Use repetition to encourage children to recognize quantity words and concepts:

△ Present songs, rhymes, words, activities, and materials multiple times, and watch for signs of familiarity.

AEPS-3 Curriculum Resources (Appendix A)

Appendix A in this volume contains numerous additional resources to supplement the AEPS-3 Curriculum. The first part of the appendix presents a list of general curriculum resources, and the second part provides lists of supplementary resources for each individual routine and activity.

AEPS-3 Skills Matrix (Appendix B)

The AEPS-3 Skills Matrix in Appendix B of this volume spotlights individual skills by showing functional application across all routines and activities. Each skills matrix (there are eight total, one for each of the test's eight developmental areas) allows you to select individual AEPS-3 items for children who require an intensive focus on a few skills across routines and activities. For children who have difficulty learning new skills at the level of individual AEPS-3 items, the Foundation Steps (*FS*) provide an even more granular breakdown of component subskills that are either a sequence of developmental precursors or steps in task analyses.

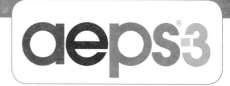

17

Meals & Snacks

Meals & Snacks can incorporate a variety of skills and provides valuable opportunities to build adult–child and peer relationships. This routine occurs frequently throughout the day, depending on the individual child and the adult. Meals & Snacks evolves over time, with infants depending completely on adults, toddlers being able to feed themselves independently, and preschoolers helping prepare meals or snacks. Through frequent repetition and growth, children acquire complex adaptive, social-communication, and fine motor skills in this routine. The AEPS-3 Beginning level of this routine uses skills from seven developmental areas.

Concurrent Skills

The following concurrent skills are AEPS-3 skills that can be easily embedded and taught during regular occurrences of Meals & Snacks.

FINE MOTOR | Beginning Skills

A 1.1   Brings hands together near midline

A 2   Grasps pea-size object

A 2.1   Grasps hand-size object

A 2.2   Grasps small cylindrical object

A 2.3   Grasps pea-size object using fingers in raking or scratching movement

A 2.4   Grasps hand-size object using whole hand

A 3   Stacks objects

B 1   Activates object with finger

B 1.1   Uses finger to point or touch

B 1.3   Uses fingers to explore object

B 2.1   Turns object using either hand

B 3.4   Holds object with one hand and manipulates object or produces action with other hand

Embedded Learning Opportunities

- *Brings hands to midline to sign MORE for more drink*
- *Takes hold of cereal pieces, crackers, or bread sticks using variety of grasps*
- *Stacks cookies on top of each other*
- *Turns empty cup in hand to indicate need for more*
- *Holds banana with one hand and animal cracker with other hand*

GROSS MOTOR Beginning Skills

A 2 Puts weight on one hand or arm while reaching with opposite hand

A 2.1 Remains propped on extended arms with head lifted

A 2.2 Remains propped on nonextended forearms with head lifted

A 4 Assumes balanced sitting position

A 4.2 Regains balanced, upright sitting position after reaching across body

A 4.3 Regains balanced, upright sitting position after leaning left, right, and forward

A 4.4 Sits balanced without support

A 4.6 Holds head in midline when sitting supported

A 5 Gets out of chair

A 5.1 Sits down in chair

A 5.2 Maintains sitting position in chair

B 1 Creeps forward using alternating arm and leg movements

B 1.3 Crawls forward on stomach

B 2 Stoops and regains balanced standing position

B 2.1 Rises from sitting to standing position

B 2.3 Pulls to standing position

B 3.1 Walks without support

B 3.2 Walks with one-hand support

B 3.3 Walks with two-hand support

B 3.4 Cruises

Embedded Learning Opportunities

- *Puts weight on one hand while sitting on floor and reaching for cracker*
- *Sits at table in child-size chair*
- *Sits in and gets up from child-size chair*
- *Crawls or creeps on picnic blanket*
- *Crawls out of booster seat after meal*
- *Walks with or without support to kitchen when food is ready*
- *Walks with or without support from outdoors to kitchen for snack*

ADAPTIVE Beginning Skills

A 1 Uses lips to take semisolid foods off eating utensil

A 1.1 Swallows semisolid foods

A 1.2 Swallows liquids

A 2.2 Eats crisp foods

A 2.3 Eats soft and dissolvable foods

A 3.2 Eats with fingers

A 3.3 Accepts food presented on eating utensils

A 4.1 Drinks from cup with spouted lid

A 4.2 Drinks from container held by adult

Embedded Learning Opportunities

- *Eats applesauce or rice cereal from eating utensil*
- *Eats crisp crackers, pretzels*
- *Drinks from spouted cup*
- *Opens mouth when adult brings spoon toward child*

SOCIAL-EMOTIONAL Beginning Skills

A 1   Initiates positive social behavior toward familiar adult

A 1.1   Responds appropriately to familiar adult's affective tone

A 1.2   Responds to familiar adult's positive social behavior

A 2   Maintains social interaction with familiar adult

A 2.1   Initiates simple social interaction with familiar adult

B 2.2   Seeks comfort, closeness, or physical contact from familiar adult

B 2.3   Responds appropriately to soothing by adult

D 4.2   Claims and defends possessions

Embedded Learning Opportunities

- *Sits in adult's lap and says "bite" when hungry*
- *Calms when adult picks up and carries child to refrigerator to get milk*
- *Responds by signing EAT when adult asks, "Are you hungry?"*
- *Says "Mama" while looking at mother and pointing to juice cup on counter*
- *Says "Mine!" when another child takes cracker*

SOCIAL-COMMUNICATION Beginning Skills

A 1   Turns and looks toward person speaking

A 1.1   Quiets to familiar voice

A 2   Produces speech sounds

A 2.1   Coos and gurgles

A 3   Engages in vocal exchanges

A 3.1   Vocalizes to another person expressing positive affective state

A 3.2   Vocalizes to another person expressing negative affective state

A 4   Uses intentional gestures, vocalizations, and objects to communicate

A 4.1   Makes requests of others

A 4.2   Makes choices to express preferences

A 4.3   Expresses desire to continue activity

A 4.4   Expresses negation or protests

B 1   Follows gaze to establish joint attention

B 1.1   Follows pointing gestures with eyes

B 1.2   Looks toward object

B 2.1   Recognizes own and familiar names

B 2.2   Responds to single-word directive

C 1.3   Uses consistent approximations for words or signs

C 1.4   Uses consistent consonant–vowel combinations

Embedded Learning Opportunities

- *Looks at adult when adult says "Here comes a bite!"*
- *Says "Mo!" when wanting more food*
- *Signs MORE or ALL DONE to communicate wants or needs*
- *Points to graham crackers when adult holds box of them and box of saltines and asks, "Which one would you like to eat?"*
- *Turns head away to protest new food*
- *Looks at object when adult asks, "What is this?" while looking toward object*
- *Sits down beside sink when adult says "Wait for me"*

COGNITIVE Beginning Skills

A 1   Orients to events or stimulation

A 1.1 Reacts to events or stimulation

A 2   Combines simple actions to examine people, animals, and objects

A 2.1 Uses sensory means to explore people, animals, and objects

B 1.1 Imitates novel simple motor action not already in repertoire

B 1.2 Imitates familiar simple motor action

B 2.1 Imitates novel vocalizations

B 2.2 Imitates familiar vocalizations

C 1.2 Locates hidden object

D 1   Uses object to obtain another object

D 1.1 Uses part of an object or support to obtain another object

D 1.2 Retains one object when second object is obtained

D 2   Coordinates actions with objects to achieve new outcomes

D 2.1 Tries different simple actions to achieve goal

D 2.2 Uses simple actions on objects

E 1.2 Uses senses to explore

E 2.3 Makes observations

Embedded Learning Opportunities

■ *Watches adult walk back and forth in kitchen while preparing food*

■ *Laughs when drops cup on floor*

■ *Mouths new foods and utensils to explore them*

■ *Tries to dry own hands after watching adult*

■ *Scoops yogurt after watching adult scoop with spoon*

■ *Locates spoon hidden under napkin*

■ *Uses spoon to get out-of-reach vegetable*

■ *Holds cracker in one hand when adult hands child second cracker for other hand*

■ *Points at flying bird during picnic and says "Look!"*

MATH Beginning Skills

A 1.2 Recites numbers 1–3

Embedded Learning Opportunities

■ *Holds up arms when adult says "1, 2, 3!" before picking up child from highchair*

◼ UNIVERSAL STRATEGIES

These are best practices for ALL young children, with attention to meeting learning outcomes within daily routines and activities of family life and early childhood classrooms while promoting positive adult–child relationships and peer interactions.

At the Beginning level of this routine, infants and young children depend on adults to supply nutritious meals and help them with the actions associated with eating. Infants begin learning skills that promote independence, such as feeding themselves and learning to drink without help. Adults should allow children to eat at their own pace, paying close attention to children's cues about satiety and hunger. It is beneficial for children to eat using their fingers in addition to being spoon fed, because it helps them develop the fine motor skills and coordination needed to eat independently. Adults can support adaptive skills by providing a wide range of age-appropriate foods with a variety of textures, flavors, smells, shapes, and colors. Consult the family doctor or pediatrician if there are questions or concerns about nutrition and eating schedules.

Interactions

Meals & Snacks at the Beginning level is a time for adult–child bonding and relationship building. Following are some suggested interactions:

▲ Include infants and children in family mealtimes whenever it is age-appropriate and in keeping with the family's customs:

△ Let young children who are not yet able to eat independently sit in a highchair and eat finger foods until an adult can feed them.

△ Let young children play with toys after eating while the rest of the family eats.

▲ Let infants and young children take food off a spoon with their lips when they start eating solid foods (adults should not push an eating utensil too far into a child's mouth, because young children have a shallow gag reflex that prevents choking). Even though it may be messy, this gives children an opportunity to learn to coordinate the muscles of their mouth and face.

▲ Allow young children adequate time to experiment with and explore new foods.

▲ Encourage young children to watch other children eat (seat them near older children or adults, if possible, so they can observe and imitate new skills).

Environment and Materials

Following are some suggestions for environment and materials at the Beginning level:

▲ Breast-feed or bottle-feed in a calm environment so the infant can focus on interacting with the adult.

▲ For children who are starting to eat solid foods,

△ Offer a variety of safe finger foods and pureed baby foods. Remember to let the child decide how much to eat.

△ Let infants and young children practice using eating utensils:

▷ Model how to hold and use the utensils to eat solid foods.

▷ Let the child try to use the utensils on their own, even if adults still end up feeding them most of the meal.

▷ Gently scaffold learning until the child can feed self independently.

▲ Provide child-size chairs or highchairs with foot rests so children's feet are supported during meals.

■ FOCUSED STRATEGIES

These strategies are for teaching SOME children who are struggling with a component of a skill or whose development is stalled and who need extra help to catch up or keep up. The strategies include a variety of minor adaptations or modifications to daily routines, activities, and environments to meet targeted outcomes at home and in classrooms.

▲ For infants who have difficulty with bottle or nipple feeding,

△ Ease swallowing by adjusting the nursing position to a more elevated but supported position.

▲ For those who have colic or who easily become overtired or hungry,

△ Keep track of the usual eating schedule and feed the child a few minutes earlier than usual, to keep them from getting distressed.

▲ For those who resist beginning solid foods,

△ Start by thinning the new food to a consistency the child will tolerate.

△ Gradually decrease the amount of liquid while increasing the amount of solid food in the mix.

▲ Keep watch for possible allergies to formula, and if allergies are present, consider changing to a soy or other alternative formula under a pediatrician's direction.

▲ Pay attention to children's cues for when they are getting hungry, and make sure mealtime occurs before they get too sleepy to participate.

▲ Remove children who become distressed at the table for a minute or two to let them calm down, and reseat them afterward if they want to come back to the table.

▲ Introduce chunky textures slowly over time using favorite foods, moving from fully pureed to a mixture containing a few small chunks.

▲ Try alleviating hypersensitive gag reflexes by using a very small spoon with a soft plastic covering.

▲ Consult parents about which eating utensils work best at home, and provide them in the classroom.

▲ Teach children who cannot speak to use simple signs (MORE, ALL DONE) so they can communicate their preferences.

▲ Learn to recognize children's cues and preferences.

▲ Pair sign language with spoken words for children who are nonverbal or who have hearing impairments.

TIER 3

■ SPECIALIZED STRATEGIES

These strategies for teaching the FEW children who need intensive supports include a variety of specialized, individualized, precise evidence-based strategies to meet children's unique goals/outcomes:

▲ Promote object labeling by using snacks and meals to teach one-word labels for favorite foods.

▲ Use the same words or signs for foods and utensils that children are used to hearing at home.

▲ For children who have vision impairments,

△ Let the child explore foods using their other senses before they try to eat.

△ Use hand-under-hand guidance to help teach utensil use.

▲ For children who have special motor or oral-motor needs,

△ Plan for extra time at meals and snacks.

△ Use hand-over-hand guidance to help older infants use utensils.

▲ For children who struggle to coordinate the suck-swallow-breathe cycle,

△ Pace feedings to prevent distress (at regular intervals, pull the nipple or bottle all or part of the way out of the child's mouth, to allow time for breathing).

△ Use a semi-reclined (partly upright) position.

△ Try a side-lying position to support coordination.

▲ For children who have support or positioning needs,

△ Use a pillow to elevate and provide extra support to keep the child's head and neck positioned properly.

△ Try seating the child on an adult's lap (or in a highchair as children get bigger), and use cushions or pillows to fill in space and keep the child comfortable.

△ Provide supportive positioning that allows children who have gross motor delays to sit completely upright to eat if they are ready for finger foods or are transitioning to solid foods.

▲ For children who have problems sucking, swallowing, chewing, or maintaining proper posture for eating,

△ Consult an occupational or physical therapist.

△ Explore the variety of specialized utensils to find ones that work best for children who have motor difficulties.

▲ For children who have extraneous tongue movements,

△ Try placing a finger underneath the bony point of the jaw.

▲ For children who experience reflux,

△ Pay particular attention to positioning after eating (typically, side-lying or partially upright and supported positions help reduce reflux).

△ Try adjusting the timing of meals (schedule smaller meals closer together throughout the day).

▲ For children who struggle to eat, have been tube fed, or have other eating-related issues that have made eating a negative experience, provide positive experiences:

△ Gently stroke the child's cheeks and mouth to provide oral stimulation.

△ Use a teething toy, pacifier, or parent's finger in the mouth.

△ Play kissing games near the child's face and mouth.

AEPS-3 Curriculum Resources (Appendix A)

Appendix A in this volume contains numerous additional resources to supplement the AEPS-3 Curriculum. The first part of the appendix presents a list of general curriculum resources, and the second part provides lists of supplementary resources for each individual routine and activity.

AEPS-3 Skills Matrix (Appendix B)

The AEPS-3 Skills Matrix in Appendix B of this volume spotlights individual skills by showing functional application across all routines and activities. Each skills matrix (there are eight total, one for each of the test's eight developmental areas) allows you to select individual AEPS-3 items for children who require an intensive focus on a few skills across routines and activities. For children who have difficulty learning new skills at the level of individual AEPS-3 items, the Foundation Steps (*FS*) provide an even more granular breakdown of component subskills that are either a sequence of developmental precursors or steps in task analyses.

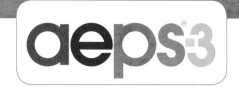

18

Music & Movement

The Music & Movement activity offers opportunities for children to learn a variety of skills in an active, social manner. This activity may include singing, dancing, participating in fingerplays, and playing musical instruments, singly or in any combination. Music and movement with infants and young children may occur one to one or in groups. This activity changes over time, with infants participating by listening to music and toddlers developing fine motor, gross motor, and communication skills that allow them to become independent participants. Children learn and acquire new skills by repeating these activities. The AEPS-3 Beginning level of Music & Movement uses skills from six developmental areas.

Concurrent Skills

The following concurrent skills are AEPS-3 skills that can be easily embedded and taught during regular occurrences of Music & Movement.

FINE MOTOR Beginning Skills

A 1   Makes directed batting or swiping movements with each hand

A 1.1   Brings hands together near midline

A 1.2   Makes directed movements with arms

A 2.1   Grasps hand-size object

A 2.2   Grasps small cylindrical object

A 3.1   Releases object into targeted space

A 3.2   Releases object into nondefined space

B 1   Activates object with finger

B 1.1   Uses finger to point or touch

B 1.2   Uses hand to activate object

B 1.3   Uses fingers to explore object

B 2.1   Turns object using either hand

B 3.4   Holds object with one hand and manipulates object or produces action with other hand

B 3.5   Transfers object from hand to hand

Embedded Learning Opportunities

- *Grasps maraca after adult shakes it*
- *Grasps instrument at midline of body*
- *Puts musical instrument back in basket after using*
- *Puts scarves back in basket after dancing with them*
- *Uses fingers to play xylophone while adult sings songs*
- *Turns knobs on music table while dancing*
- *Holds music stick in one hand and hits it with stick in other hand*

GROSS MOTOR Beginning Skills

A 1   Turns head, moves arms, and kicks legs independently of each other

A 1.1   Kicks legs

A 1.2   Waves arms

A 1.3   Turns head side to side

A 4   Assumes balanced sitting position

A 4.1   Assumes hands-and-knees position from sitting

A 4.2   Regains balanced, upright sitting position after reaching across body

A 4.3   Regains balanced, upright sitting position after leaning left, right, and forward

A 4.4   Sits balanced without support

A 4.5   Sits balanced using hands for support

A 4.6   Holds head in midline when sitting supported

B 2   Stoops and regains balanced standing position

B 2.1   Rises from sitting to standing position

B 2.2   Stands unsupported

B 2.3   Pulls to standing position

B 3.1   Walks without support

B 3.2   Walks with one-hand support

B 3.3   Walks with two-hand support

Embedded Learning Opportunities

■ *Explores body movements during movement activities while adult sings and helps*

■ *Observes movement before imitating*

■ *Balances while seated to reach for and grasp instruments out of reach*

■ *Bends down and touches toes while imitating yoga movements*

■ *Rises from sitting position to participate in Ring Around the Rosie*

■ *Walks in circle to follow marching adult*

SOCIAL-EMOTIONAL Beginning Skills

A 1   Initiates positive social behavior toward familiar adult

A 1.1   Responds appropriately to familiar adult's affective tone

A 1.2   Responds to familiar adult's positive social behavior

A 2   Maintains social interaction with familiar adult

A 2.1   Initiates simple social interaction with familiar adult

A 2.2   Repeats part of interactive game or action in order to continue game or action

B 2.2   Seeks comfort, closeness, or physical contact from familiar adult

B 2.3   Responds appropriately to soothing by adult

C 1.3   Plays near one or two peers

D 4.2   Claims and defends possessions

Embedded Learning Opportunities

■ *Smiles when hears adult singing*

■ *Asks for more songs when adult stops singing*

■ *Starts "Head, Shoulders, Knees, and Toes" movements to make adult sing it*

■ *Anticipates actions when singing Pat-a-cake*

■ *Calms down when adult says "It will be okay"*

■ *Sits next to peers while playing instruments*

■ *Dances next to peers*

■ *Holds on to drum and says "No!" when peer touches it*

SOCIAL-COMMUNICATION Beginning Skills

A 1   Turns and looks toward person speaking

A 1.1   Quiets to familiar voice

A 2   Produces speech sounds

A 2.1   Coos and gurgles

A 3   Engages in vocal exchanges

A 3.1   Vocalizes to another person expressing positive affective state

A 3.2   Vocalizes to another person expressing negative affective state

A 4   Uses intentional gestures, vocalizations, and objects to communicate

A 4.1   Makes requests of others

A 4.2   Makes choices to express preferences

A 4.3   Expresses desire to continue activity

A 4.4   Expresses negation or protests

B 1   Follows gaze to establish joint attention

B 1.1   Follows pointing gestures with eyes

B 1.2   Looks toward object

B 2.1   Recognizes own and familiar names

B 2.2   Responds to single-word directive

C 1.3   Uses consistent approximations for words or signs

C 1.4   Uses consistent consonant–vowel combinations

Embedded Learning Opportunities

■ *Looks at adult singing*

■ *Vocalizes speechlike sounds in response to being sung to*

■ *Laughs when adult sings silly songs*

■ *Says "No!" when adult starts singing song child does not want*

■ *Asks, "Bus?" to sing "Wheels on the Bus"*

■ *Signs MORE or ALL DONE to continue or cease music*

■ *Claps hands together after music stops in anticipation of more music*

■ *Looks up at sky when adult points up to sky during movement*

■ *Looks at material (puppet, scarf, instrument) when adult looks at material and says "What is that?"*

■ *Claps when adult says "Clap!"*

■ *Says "tink, tink" when singing "Twinkle, Twinkle, Little Star"*

COGNITIVE Beginning Skills

A 1   Orients to events or stimulation

A 1.1   Reacts to events or stimulation

A 2   Combines simple actions to examine people, animals, and objects

A 2.1   Uses sensory means to explore people, animals, and objects

B 1.1   Imitates novel simple motor action not already in repertoire

B 1.2   Imitates familiar simple motor action

B 2.1   Imitates novel vocalizations

B 2.2   Imitates familiar vocalizations

E 1.2   Uses senses to explore

E 2.3   Makes observations

Embedded Learning Opportunities

■ *Turns head to follow or look for sound*

■ *Dances to sound of music*

■ *Examines new instruments before shaking*

■ *Mouths instruments during music*

■ *Bangs on drum for first time after adult or peer models*

■ *Says "ra-ra" after adult sings "Roar, roar, dinosaur!"*

■ *Says "Yay!" after adult says "Yay! Great dancing!"*

■ *Says "Loud!" when adult turns music up*

MATH Beginning Skills

A 1.2   Recites numbers 1–3

TIER 1

■ UNIVERSAL STRATEGIES

These are best practices for ALL young children, with attention to meeting learning outcomes within daily routines and activities of family life and early childhood classrooms while promoting positive adult-child relationships and peer interactions.

Music and movement for infants and young children at the Beginning level incorporates a variety of skills in many developmental areas. Through both music and movement, infants learn transitions, language, rhythm, play skills, names, listening skills, and bonding. Adults can support learning through music and movement by providing a range of experiences throughout the day and incorporating them into everyday experiences.

Interactions

Through music, children learn to match the sounds of language by listening to and repeating songs. In particular, songs that use gestures or objects help children begin to develop language comprehension. Infants learn listening skills by learning to follow along with words and directions. Adult-child bonding also occurs when an adult sings to an infant and the infant finds joy and comfort in the adult's voice. Following are some suggested interactions for the Beginning level of this routine:

▲ Use music and songs to help make transitions more predictable during daily routines (sing waking, diapering, or sleeping songs).

▲ Use music to help infants learn new words, word sounds, and communication.

▲ Involve other children or siblings in music and movement, both to serve as models and to help infants build relationships with others.

Environment and Materials

Environments that are rich in music and movement encourage infants to explore and experiment with words, language, and rhythm. Following are some suggestions for environment and materials at the Beginning level:

▲ Allow time for children to interact with a variety of developmentally appropriate instruments or sound makers to help them learn about volume (loud and quiet), rate (fast and slow), and following directions (go and stop).

▲ Play child-appropriate music that includes children's interests.

▲ Use songs with catchy tunes and easy-to-learn lyrics to help children learn rhythm and language.

▲ Use songs with children's names in them, because children love to hear their own name.

▲ Use a variety of music from different cultures, genres, and styles.

▲ Incorporate simple gross or fine motor opportunities to let children use trial and error while exploring how their bodies move.

■ FOCUSED STRATEGIES

These strategies are for teaching SOME children who are struggling with a component of a skill or whose development is stalled and who need extra help to catch up or keep up. The strategies include a variety of minor adaptations or modifications to daily routines, activities, and environments to meet targeted outcomes at home and in classrooms.

▲ Offer opportunities during multiple daily routines for children to hear and engage with music, fingerplays, movement, and musical instruments.

▲ Pay close attention for times when babies are comfortable, alert, and ready to learn or play, and take advantage of them as opportunities for music and movement.

▲ Use repetition to encourage children to engage in rhyming and rhythm and trying out new words and movements.

▲ Make sure to present songs, rhymes, words, activities, and materials multiple times, and watch for signs of familiarity. Some children may take a while to warm up to new materials or games and may need many opportunities to watch and observe before they participate.

▲ Introduce children to rhymes and songs that use their fingers and toes. When children seem able to anticipate and engage with simple gestures and words, expand on the actions or start learning a new song.

▲ Engage older toddlers or siblings in presenting musical instruments to infants or singing to them, because infants may be reluctant to interact with less familiar adults.

▲ Give children who have a hard time sitting and listening to music a fidget toy or something to hold (may help them engage).

▲ Teach children who cannot speak to use simple signs (MORE, ALL DONE) so they can communicate their preferences.

▲ Learn to recognize children's cues and preferences.

▲ Pair sign language with spoken words for children who are nonverbal or who have hearing impairments.

■ SPECIALIZED STRATEGIES

These strategies for teaching the FEW children who need intensive supports include a variety of specialized, individualized, precise evidence-based strategies to meet children's unique goals/outcomes:

▲ Integrate music into soothing activities (rocking, rubbing a child's back before nap) for children who have limited periods of attention and engagement.

▲ Use hand-over-hand assistance to help children clap rhythm with music or learn a new musical instrument:

△ Use most-to-least prompting to fade hand-over-hand assistance.

△ Move physical prompting from hands, to wrists, to forearms.

▲ For children who have vision impairments,

△ Use tangible items that relate to the songs being sung.

▲ For children who have hearing impairments,

△ Pair music with visual cues such as flashing lights or vibration.

▲ For children who have vision and/or hearing impairments,

△ Seat the singer or movement leader close by.

AEPS-3 Curriculum Resources (Appendix A)

Appendix A in this volume contains numerous additional resources to supplement the AEPS-3 Curriculum. The first part of the appendix presents a list of general curriculum resources, and the second part provides lists of supplementary resources for each individual routine and activity.

AEPS-3 Skills Matrix (Appendix B)

The AEPS-3 Skills Matrix in Appendix B of this volume spotlights individual skills by showing functional application across all routines and activities. Each skills matrix (there are eight total, one for each of the test's eight developmental areas) allows you to select individual AEPS-3 items for children who require an intensive focus on a few skills across routines and activities. For children who have difficulty learning new skills at the level of individual AEPS-3 items, the Foundation Steps (*FS*) provide an even more granular breakdown of component subskills that are either a sequence of developmental precursors or steps in task analyses.

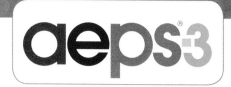

19

Nap & Sleep

Nap & Sleep can occur in any environment, and very young children may sleep several times a day. The number of times infants sleep daily and the number of hours needed generally decrease as children grow. This routine changes over time as children's adaptive, cognitive, social-emotional, and motor skills develop.

Sleep is critical for children to stay healthy and regulated. Infants depend completely on adults to support their need for sleep, and to do so, adults must notice and interpret a variety of sometimes subtle verbal and nonverbal cues. Facial expressions, patterns of attention and activity, and the quality of an infant's crying can all indicate a need for sleep. As a rule, sleepy babies should not be challenged to perform difficult tasks or learn new skills. The AEPS-3 Beginning level of this routine uses skills from seven developmental areas.

Concurrent Skills

The following concurrent skills are AEPS-3 skills that can be easily embedded and taught during regular occurrences of Nap & Sleep.

FINE MOTOR Beginning Skills

A 1   Makes directed batting or swiping movements with each hand

A 1.2   Makes directed movements with arms

B 1.1   Uses finger to point or touch

B 1.2   Uses hand to activate object

B 3.5   Transfers object from hand to hand

Embedded Learning Opportunities

- *Plays with mobile hanging over crib*

- *Points to crib or bed to indicate readiness for sleep*

- *Activates musical toy to listen to while falling asleep*

GROSS MOTOR Beginning Skills

A 1.3 Turns head side to side

A 3   Rolls from back to stomach

A 3.1 Rolls from stomach to back

A 3.2 Rolls from back or stomach to side

B 2.3 Pulls to standing position

B 2.4 Pulls to kneeling position

B 3.1 Walks without support

B 3.2 Walks with one-hand support

B 3.3 Walks with two-hand support

Embedded Learning Opportunities

■ *Moves body around in crib or bed by rolling to get comfortable*

■ *Uses crib rail to pull up to knees or feet upon waking*

■ *Walks with or without support on nature walk with adult*

ADAPTIVE Beginning Skills

A 1.2 Swallows liquids

A 4.1 Drinks from cup with spouted lid

A 4.2 Drinks from container held by adult

C 1.5 Takes off shoes

C 1.6 Takes off socks

Embedded Learning Opportunities

■ *Drinks from bottle or cup held by adult as part of naptime routine*

■ *Takes off socks and shoes to prepare for nap*

SOCIAL EMOTIONAL Beginning Skills

A 1   Initiates positive social behavior toward familiar adult

A 1.1 Responds appropriately to familiar adult's affective tone

A 2.1 Initiates simple social interaction with familiar adult

B 2.2 Seeks comfort, closeness, physical contact from familiar adult

B 2.3 Responds appropriately to soothing by adult

Embedded Learning Opportunities

■ *Goes to or calls for adult for comfort and closeness when trying to fall asleep*

■ *Smiles and is soothed by adult singing lullaby or reading book*

SOCIAL COMMUNICATION Beginning Skills

A 1.1 Quiets to familiar voice

A 4.1 Makes requests of others

A 4.2 Makes choices to express preferences

A 4.4 Expresses negation or protests

C 1.3 Uses consistent approximations for words or signs

C 1.4 Uses consistent consonant-vowel combinations

Embedded Learning Opportunities

■ *Stops crying upon hearing adult's voice after waking*

■ *Brings book to adult to indicate desire to read*

■ *Shakes head side to side to indicate does not want to sleep*

■ *Says "ni-ni" for good night when going to bed*

LITERACY Beginning Skills

A 1.1 Participates in shared one-on-one reading

Embedded Learning Opportunities

■ *Listens to adult reading story before nap or bedtime*

MATH Beginning Skills

A 1.2 Recites numbers 1–3

Embedded Learning Opportunities

■ *Counts "1, 2, 3" before getting picked up out of crib*

TIER 1

■ UNIVERSAL STRATEGIES

These are best practices for ALL young children, with attention to meeting learning outcomes within daily routines and activities of family life and early childhood classrooms while promoting positive adult–child relationships and peer interactions.

Nap and sleep routines for infants may vary greatly, but in general, very young children transition quickly between states of sleeping and waking. They may be sound asleep one minute and then wide awake and crying after a loud noise. Some drowsy infants can fall asleep independently after being placed in their cribs, but many need help by being rocked, patted, sung to, or read to sleep. Through nap and sleep routines, infants and young children can learn techniques to calm their bodies when drowsy. Naptime should be based on children's needs but should also occur at a similar time each day to promote a consistent schedule (younger infants will sleep after every feeding, whereas older infants and young toddlers may need only one nap each day). For some children, the best nap time may be directly after lunch, whereas for others, it may be midmorning or midafternoon. Consistency and predictability will help children develop the self-soothing skills needed to fall asleep easily.

Interactions

Rest times for infants and young children present opportunities for adult–child bonding and relationship building. Following are some suggested interactions for the Beginning level of Nap & Sleep:

▲ Promote bonding:

△ Become familiar with infants' unique sleep patterns, and respond to cues that they are getting drowsy. Recognize that it may take time for infants to develop a regular sleep-wake cycle.

△ Keep rest time routines consistent.

△ Respond quickly to any needs that arise during this routine.

▲ Help young children relax and feel comfortable so they can fall asleep more easily:

△ Follow a consistent, familiar routine both at home and in child care settings.

△ Read favorite books and sing calming songs while holding, rocking, or patting the child.

△ Make sure the child has a full stomach to promote drowsiness and longer sleep (eating and sleeping are closely associated in infants).

△ Provide a suitable sleep environment.

Environment and Materials

Following are some suggestions for environment and materials for the Beginning level of this routine:

▲ Establish a familiar sleep environment for young infants and children. They will rest most easily when they have a consistent place to sleep (in a child care setting, always place infants in the same crib, and always set young toddlers' cots in the same spots in the classroom).

▲ Dim the lights and provide gentle background noise (sound machine, lullaby music) to help keep noise distractions to a minimum.

▲ Take steps to minimize the risk of sudden infant death syndrome (SIDS) and suffocation:

△ Lay infants on their back to sleep.

△ Keep cribs clear of blankets, pillows, plush toys, and crib bumpers.

△ Provide firm mattresses for infants to sleep on, or use a sleep sack if desired. Do not use soft mattresses.

△ Make sure all cribs and cots used for sleeping meet all minimum safety requirements.

TIER 2

■ FOCUSED STRATEGIES

These strategies are for teaching SOME children who are struggling with a component of a skill or whose development is stalled and who need extra help to catch up or keep up. The strategies include a variety of minor adaptations or modifications to daily routines, activities, and environments to meet targeted outcomes at home and in classrooms.

▲ Provide the opportunity for napping when children are most ready. They will likely be more resistant to sleep when they have just finished an exciting activity or are generally not sleepy.

▲ Read books about bedtime to help children understand the routine.

▲ Sing songs or read books children enjoy to encourage their willing participation in sleep routines.

▲ Consider offering thinned solid food (a bit of baby cereal in milk) in the evening for children who have problems going to sleep and staying asleep.

▲ Help infants who need assistance in calming their bodies for rest:

△ Rock, pat, sing, or read to the child until they are drowsy or (for some) until they fall asleep.

△ Pat and sing a child to sleep after they are in their bed or crib to avoid moving them once they are drowsy or in a light sleep state.

▲ Take the time in home programs to talk to family caregivers about sleep routines at home and specific problems children have (falling asleep, staying asleep), working together to identify specific approaches that are acceptable to the family.

▲ Start the routine earlier for infants who need more soothing and calming before falling asleep.

▲ Learn to recognize children's cues and preferences.

▲ Teach children who cannot speak to use simple signs (MORE, ALL DONE) so they can communicate their preferences.

▲ Pair sign language with spoken words for children who are nonverbal or who have hearing impairments.

■ SPECIALIZED STRATEGIES

These strategies for teaching the FEW children who need intensive supports include a variety of specialized, individualized, precise evidence-based strategies to meet children's unique goals/outcomes:

▲ Accommodate specific physical or medical needs:

   △ Provide adapted sleep equipment (wedges, hammocks) as necessary.

   △ Make sure all adaptations have been written up and approved by a physician or physical therapist.

▲ For children who have difficulty calming down for sleep,

   △ Use positive reinforcement by letting the child choose a soft toy from a basket when lying appropriately on a cot.

   △ Fade calming that relies on an adult's physical presence:

      ▷ Put the child in the crib or on the cot and walk away.

      ▷ Wait a specified amount of time. If the child has not calmed down to go to sleep by that point, only then go back to help.

      ▷ Gradually increase the amount of wait time before going back.

      ▷ Move from physical calming (rubbing, patting) to verbal calming (singing, soothing voice). Then fade verbal calming from using your voice next to the crib to using it at the bedroom door.

AEPS-3 Curriculum Resources (Appendix A)

Appendix A in this volume contains numerous additional resources to supplement the AEPS-3 Curriculum. The first part of the appendix presents a list of general curriculum resources, and the second part provides lists of supplementary resources for each individual routine and activity.

AEPS-3 Skills Matrix (Appendix B)

The AEPS-3 Skills Matrix in Appendix B of this volume spotlights individual skills by showing functional application across all routines and activities. Each skills matrix (there are eight total, one for each of the test's eight developmental areas) allows you to select individual AEPS-3 items for children who require an intensive focus on a few skills across routines and activities. For children who have difficulty learning new skills at the level of individual AEPS-3 items, the Foundation Steps (FS) provide an even more granular breakdown of component subskills that are either a sequence of developmental precursors or steps in task analyses.

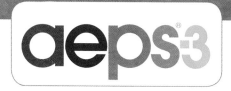

20

Sensory

The Sensory activity offers opportunities for children to learn and explore a variety of materials through play, investigation, exploration, and sensory processes to develop touch, smell, taste, sight, and hearing skills. Sensory play encourages children to manipulate materials, explore surfaces, lift, throw, roll, and pour, and it can take place in a variety of settings (sensory table, highchair, bathtub).

This activity evolves over time as children's cognitive, communication, social-emotional, and motor skills increase and as children shift from exploring common items (toys, blankets and fabrics, food containers, food) to more advanced materials (playdough, sand and dirt, chewable food items, dried beans). The AEPS-3 Beginning level of Sensory uses skills from eight developmental areas.

Concurrent Skills

The following concurrent skills are AEPS-3 skills that can be easily embedded and taught during regular occurrences of Sensory.

FINE MOTOR Beginning Skills

A 1.2   Makes directed movements with arms

A 2.1   Grasps hand-size object

A 2.2   Grasps small cylindrical object

A 2.3   Grasps pea-size object using fingers in raking or scratching movement

A 2.4   Grasps hand-size object using whole hand

A 3.1   Releases object into targeted space

A 3.2   Releases object into nondefined space

B 1   Activates object with finger

B 1.1   Uses finger to point or touch

B 1.3   Uses fingers to explore object

B 2.1   Turns object with either hand

B 3.4   Holds object with one hand and manipulates object or produces action with other hand

B 3.5   Transfers object from hand to hand

Embedded Learning Opportunities

- *Scoops sand and water in sensory table and pours back into table or container (bucket)*

- *Uses fingers and hands to explore, manipulate, and transfer materials with variety of textures (sand, water, mulch, grass, playdough)*

- *Uses one finger to turn on electronic musical toy*

- *Turns bottle to look at liquid and materials inside (glitter)*

- *Holds tambourine with one hand while hitting it with other hand to make sound*

GROSS MOTOR Beginning Skills

A 1   Turns head, moves arms, and kicks legs independently of each other

A 1.3 Turns head side to side

A 2   Puts weight on one hand or arm while reaching with opposite hand

A 2.1 Remains propped on extended arms with head lifted

A 2.2 Remains propped on nonextended forearms with head lifted

A 4   Assumes balanced sitting position

A 4.1 Assumes hands-and-knees position from sitting

A 4.2 Regains balanced, upright sitting position after reaching across body

A 4.3 Regains balanced, upright sitting position after leaning left, right, and forward

A 4.4 Sits balanced without support

A 4.6 Holds head in midline when sitting supported

B 1.3 Crawls forward on stomach

B 1.4 Pivots on stomach

B 2   Stoops and regains balanced standing position

B 2.1 Rises from sitting to standing position

B 2.2 Stands unsupported

B 2.3 Pulls to standing position

B 2.4 Pulls to kneeling position

C 1.6 Throws or rolls ball at target with two hands

Embedded Learning Opportunities

■ *Lies or sits on play mat with toys and materials of a variety of textures within reach (bumpy balls, crinkle toys)*

■ *Uses motor skills to reach for and examine materials on water play mat*

■ *Holds head at midline or turns head side to side while in upright seated position to watch bubbles float*

■ *Crawls or walks barefoot on surfaces with different textures (grass, carpet)*

■ *Pulls up to or stands at sensory table during sand or water play*

■ *Throws small snowball, ball of kinetic sand, or ball of playdough overhead*

ADAPTIVE Beginning Skills

A 2.2 Eats crisp foods

A 2.3 Eats soft and dissolvable foods

A 3.2 Eats with fingers

Embedded Learning Opportunities

■ *Uses fingers to eat variety of foods of different temperatures*

■ *Eats applesauce on rice cracker with fingers*

SOCIAL-EMOTIONAL Beginning Skills

B 2.2 Seeks comfort, closeness, or physical contact from familiar adult

B 2.3 Responds appropriately to soothing by adult

C 1.3 Plays near one or two peers

Embedded Learning Opportunities

■ *Allows self to be soothed by adult when uncomfortable during sensory experience (loud siren, fire alarm)*

■ *Plays beside peer during activity (group finger painting)*

SOCIAL-COMMUNICATION Beginning Skills

A 1   Turns and looks toward person speaking

A 2   Produces speech sounds

A 2.1 Coos and gurgles

A 3   Engages in vocal exchanges

A 3.1 Vocalizes to another person expressing positive affective state

A 3.2 Vocalizes to another person expressing negative affective state

A 4   Uses intentional gestures, vocalizations, and objects to communicate

A 4.2 Makes choices to express preferences

A 4.3 Expresses desire to continue activity

A 4.4 Expresses negation or protests

B 1.2 Looks toward object

C 1.3 Uses consistent word approximations for words or signs

Embedded Learning Opportunities

■ *Hears person speaking or object making noise and looks in that direction*

■ *Vocalizes or gestures to express enjoyment or discomfort during activity (sand and water play)*

■ *Says "no" for snow; "bud" for bird, "wa" for water upon seeing those things*

COGNITIVE Beginning Skills

A 1   Orients to events or stimulation

A 1.1 Reacts to events or stimulation

A 2   Combines simple actions to examine people, animals, and objects

A 2.1 Uses sensory means to explore people, animals, and objects

D 1.2 Retains one object when second object is obtained

D 2   Coordinates actions with objects to achieve new outcomes

D 2.2 Uses simple actions on objects

E 1.2 Uses senses to explore

E 2.3 Makes observations

Embedded Learning Opportunities

■ *Turns head or body to orient and react to noise-producing object (rain stick, toy drum, rattle)*

■ *Holds objects (ball, rattle, block) in hands and drops them to explore result*

■ *Explores variety of objects through senses (mouthing, touching, listening) to get acquainted with them*

LITERACY Beginning Skills

A 1.1 Participates in shared one-on-one reading

Embedded Learning Opportunities

■ *Sits in adult's lap and engages with touch book by feeling and looking at book*

MATH Beginning Skills

A 1.2   Recites numbers 1-3

Embedded Learning Opportunities

- *Counts to 3 when hitting tambourine, shaking a rattle, or hitting music sticks together*

TIER 1

■ UNIVERSAL STRATEGIES

These are best practices for ALL young children, with attention to meeting learning outcomes within daily routines and activities of family life and early childhood classrooms while promoting positive adult–child relationships and peer interactions.

During all routines and activities, infants and young children learn primarily through sensory exploration. For infants, sensory learning is an important way they explore their environment. They begin learning about the world around them through textures, tastes, sounds, sights, and smells. Infants must learn how to orient to auditory and visual stimuli in order to acquire practical communication skills and develop information processing and social interaction. For young children, tactile sensitivity alerts them to extreme temperatures and pain, thus helping them avoid physical danger and maintain good health. They learn basic sensorimotor skills by locating, orienting, and responding to a variety of social and nonsocial objects in the environment and to auditory, visual, and tactile events.

It is important and beneficial for adults to provide children with a variety of textures, sounds, sights, tastes, and smells within their environment:

▲ Hang pictures and art in the classroom at a level children are able to see.

▲ Describe classroom objects (art, other items) to children to teach descriptive words that help build vocabulary.

▲ Make available a variety of developmentally appropriate toys for children to manipulate and examine through touch.

▲ Hang a sensory board low on the wall to provide opportunities to feel a variety of textures (rough, soft, bumpy, smooth, slippery) all in one location and help children learn about similarities and differences of materials in their environment.

▲ Make teething toys and rattles accessible for children to mouth, as these provide a lot of sensory input.

▲ Wash and sanitize toys properly after each time children mouth them, to prevent the spread of illness.

Interactions

Take advantage of the sensory interactions that occur constantly with young children in their natural environments. Following are some suggestions for the Beginning level of this activity:

▲ Use different voice intonations while talking with or singing to children to provide sensory experience through sound.

▲ Encourage children to try foods with a variety of textures, tastes, and temperatures at mealtimes.

▲ Describe foods to children using words like *sweet, salty, warm,* and *cold* to help them become aware of differences among foods they eat.

▲ Incorporate opportunities for sensory input by encouraging children to explore a variety of textures using materials at home or in the classroom (bumpy balls, smooth blocks, textured blocks, warm water, cold water, ice packs, soft towels, paper).

Environment and Materials

Following are some suggestions for providing sensory experiences for children at the Beginning level:

▲ Encourage infants to turn, look, reach for, or move toward visual stimuli within their visual field that do not produce sound.

▲ Give children noise-producing objects to manipulate (rattle, crinkly paper).

▲ Help children learn to differentiate between sounds and silence (speak and then pause; turn on the radio, then shut it off and wait for the child to respond).

▲ Stop the activity that is occurring and encourage children to listen to the sounds in the environment (dogs barking, children shouting, appliances running, airplanes flying over).

▲ Take children to find the noises they hear.

▲ Hide yourself or a toy and continue speaking or making noise with the toy.

▲ Teach infants to differentiate among sensory stimuli by alternating low tones (such as those made with wooden objects) with high tones (made with plastic objects) and loud sounds (singing) with soft sounds (whispering).

▲ Attach noise-producing objects to children's arms or legs (jingle bells on socks or wrist).

▲ Help children learn to track, turn their heads, reach, and maintain visual contact by slowly moving objects they are focusing on visually.

▲ Determine which cues infants respond to and orient toward most readily by

△ Using a variety of colors and patterns over time

△ Beginning with a few cues and gradually presenting others until the infant can generalize the skill across a variety of visual cues

▲ Hold objects directly in children's visual field, at a distance where visual clarity is best.

▲ Use large, brightly colored objects or objects with patterned surfaces, in play, to capture children's attention.

▲ Give children materials that stick to their fingers (cereal, playdough, finger paint), and wipe their hands clean afterward, to let them experience different textures.

▲ Vary the textures of tactile cues over time to determine which cues children respond and orient to most readily.

▲ Make sure all sensory items are developmentally appropriate and safe for infants.

▲ Make sure adults are always present during sensory routines.

TIER 2

■ FOCUSED STRATEGIES

These strategies are for teaching SOME children who are struggling with a component of a skill or whose development is stalled and who need extra help to catch up or keep up. The strategies include a variety of minor adaptations or modifications to daily routines, activities, and environments to meet targeted outcomes at home and in classrooms.

▲ Allow children to engage in a variety of sensory activities (tactile, visual, sound, taste) by incorporating opportunities into multiple daily routines.

▲ Use verbal and physical prompts to help children become active participants in sensory activities.

▲ Introduce new sensory materials and activities slowly, allowing time for children to become comfortable with one before moving on to another.

▲ Offer children who are particularly sensitive (or insensitive) to a particular type of sensory experience more frequent exposures to that experience to gradually ease the child into more intense experiences.

▲ Offer sensory experiences in a variety of settings to help children generalize those experiences through repetition.

▲ Teach children who cannot speak to use simple signs (MORE, ALL DONE) so they can communicate their preferences.

▲ Learn to recognize children's cues and preferences.

▲ Pair sign language with spoken words for children who are nonverbal or who have hearing impairments.

■ SPECIALIZED STRATEGIES

These strategies for teaching the FEW children who need intensive supports include a variety of specialized, individualized, precise evidence-based strategies to meet children's unique goals/outcomes:

▲ Embed a variety of sensory materials into various routines throughout the day for children who have limited attention and engagement:

△ At mealtime, touch a warm bottle to the infant's skin.

△ For rest time, place a mobile near the crib or play soothing music.

△ At reading time, use touch-and-feel books.

▲ Provide hand-over-hand assistance to help children become active participants in sensory activities; use graduated guidance to slowly fade the assistance.

▲ Offer children who are blind or who have other visual impairments multiple opportunities to have tactile or auditory sensory experiences:

△ Use hand-<u>under</u>-hand prompting if needed.

△ Label all sensory experiences verbally.

▲ Offer children who are deaf or who have other hearing impairments multiple opportunities to have visual or tactile sensory experiences, using total communication (verbal and signed) to label sensory stimuli.

▲ Keep materials and activities short and simple for children who become easily overwhelmed or overstimulated, and provide comfort and closeness to make the activity more tolerable.

AEPS-3 Curriculum Resources (Appendix A)

Appendix A in this volume contains numerous additional resources to supplement the AEPS-3 Curriculum. The first part of the appendix presents a list of general curriculum resources, and the second part provides lists of supplementary resources for each individual routine and activity.

AEPS-3 Skills Matrix (Appendix B)

The AEPS-3 Skills Matrix in Appendix B of this volume spotlights individual skills by showing functional application across all routines and activities. Each skills matrix (there are eight total, one for each of the test's eight developmental areas) allows you to select individual AEPS-3 items for children who require an intensive focus on a few skills across routines and activities. For children who have difficulty learning new skills at the level of individual AEPS-3 items, the Foundation Steps (FS) provide an even more granular breakdown of component subskills that are either a sequence of developmental precursors or steps in task analyses.

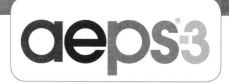

21

Writing

The Writing activity changes over time as infants develop more refined skills related to the activity. The elements of writing vary and include materials, media, location (indoors and outdoors), participants, and use of children's creativity and imagination to create projects. Writing activities at the Beginning level can take place in the home or at child care, in small groups or individually. Writing is not limited to pencil on paper but can also include crayons, chalk, markers, paint brushes, and finger paints. Writing changes across skill areas as children's motor, cognitive, communication, and social-emotional skills increase, and the routine can address a number of developmental skills. Young children start writing by first making marks on a surface; then scribbling; then making horizontal, vertical, and diagonal lines; and finally transitioning to forming letters, numbers, and words. The AEPS-3 Beginning level of this routine uses skills from seven developmental areas.

Concurrent Skills

The following concurrent skills are AEPS-3 skills that can be easily embedded and taught during regular occurrences of Writing.

FINE MOTOR Beginning Skills

A 2.1 Grasps hand-size object
A 2.2 Grasps small cylindrical object
B 1.1 Uses finger to point or touch
B 1.3 Uses fingers to explore object
B 3.5 Transfers object from hand to hand

Embedded Learning Opportunities

- *Grasps jumbo marker, crayon, paintbrush, chalk*
- *Uses fingers to create and explore finger paint*
- *Transfers marker, crayon, paintbrush, chalk from one hand to other*

GROSS MOTOR Beginning Skills

A 4   Assumes balanced sitting position
A 4.4 Sits balanced without support
A 5   Gets out of chair
A 5.1 Sits down in chair
A 5.2 Maintains sitting position in chair
B 3.1 Walks without support
B 3.2 Walks with one-hand support
B 3.3 Walks with two-hand support

Embedded Learning Opportunities

- *Sits on towel or sheet while drawing with sidewalk chalk*
- *Sits down on and gets out of chair to draw with markers or crayons*
- *Walks with or without support from bedroom to kitchen where art supplies are set out*

SOCIAL-EMOTIONAL Beginning Skills

C 1.3 Plays near one or two peers
D 3.3 Entertains self by playing with toys
D 4.2 Claims and defends possessions

Embedded Learning Opportunities

■ *Participates in group finger painting activity*

■ *Plays on own by making dots with marker or finger paint*

■ *Holds onto marker when another child tries to take it*

SOCIAL-COMMUNICATION Beginning Skills

A 2   Produces speech sounds
A 4.2 Makes choices to express preferences
B 1   Follows gaze to establish joint attention
B 1.1 Follows pointing gestures with eyes
B 1.2 Looks toward object
C 1.3 Uses consistent approximations for words or signs
C 1.4 Uses consistent consonant–vowel combinations

Embedded Learning Opportunities

■ *Uses speech sounds, vocalizations, or word approximations to imitate color words*

■ *Looks toward container of crayons or markers that adult is pointing to and looking at*

■ *Chooses marker, crayon, or piece of chalk from container*

COGNITIVE Beginning Skills

B 1.1 Imitates novel simple motor action not already in repertoire
B 1.2 Imitates familiar simple motor action
D 1   Uses object to obtain another object
D 1.1 Uses part of object or support to obtain another object
E 1.2 Uses senses to explore
E 2.3 Makes observations

Embedded Learning Opportunities

■ *Uses dot marker by banging it on paper after adult models action*

■ *Uses jumbo marker to pull another marker to self*

■ *Makes scribbles and dots with markers to observe difference in marks made*

LITERACY Beginning Skills

A 1.1 Participates in shared one-on-one reading

Embedded Learning Opportunities

■ *Listens to adult read book before writing activity, and participates by looking at and pointing to pictures*

MATH Beginning Skills

A 1.2   Recites numbers 1–3

Embedded Learning Opportunities

■ *Says "1, 2, 3" after adult makes three marks on paper and counts to 3*

TIER 1

■ UNIVERSAL STRATEGIES

These are best practices for ALL young children, with attention to meeting learning outcomes within daily routines and activities of family life and early childhood classrooms while promoting positive adult–child relationships and peer interactions.

The foundation for writing skills comes from overall fine motor development. The following practices help infants and young children develop the fine motor skills necessary for writing:

▲ Offer a variety of fine motor materials and activities.

▲ Encourage very young infants to reach for and hold on to rattles to help develop their ability to grasp hand-size objects.

▲ Introduce more challenging fine motor activities as infants' fine motor skills progress.

Interactions

Following are some suggested interactions for the Beginning level of Writing:

▲ Encourage children to explore and develop fine motor skills by giving them a variety of developmentally appropriate materials they can manipulate and use to build strength in their hands.

▲ Model how different writing media work while allowing children to be creative and experiment.

▲ Use descriptive language while infants experiment with various media ("You used lots of colors! I see green, red, and blue!")

▲ Always supervise young children's use of writing media.

Environment and Materials

Writing activities can take place in many different environments, including home, school, and outdoors. When older infants and young toddlers are ready, it is important to provide them with opportunities to practice scribbling with a variety of different writing and drawing materials. Following are some suggestions for the Beginning level of the Writing routine:

▲ Offer a variety of developmentally appropriate writing and drawing materials to help develop fine motor skills:

   △ Provide puzzles with knobs, shape sorters, pop-up boxes, small blocks, and manipulatives.

   △ Provide nontoxic, washable, chunky writing media such as crayons, markers, and paints.

△ Provide paintbrushes, crayons, chalk, and markers in chunky versions suitable for beginners, which young toddlers often find easier to grasp when they are learning how to scribble.

△ Let young children use markers, crayons, dot markers, chalk, and paintbrushes as often as possible to help them develop refined writing skills.

▲ Provide washable materials to save on cleanup, because infants who are learning to scribble have little control over where their writing media go.

▲ Supply clothing protectors such as plastic paint smocks or old clothes.

▲ Place a painting tarp, newspaper, or piece of plastic on the floor to protect it; avoid slipping and tripping hazards when placing floor coverings.

▲ Define spaces where children can keep their writing media by using trays or taping straws to the edge of a piece of paper.

▲ Incorporate writing-related activities at home:

△ Offer supervised opportunities to use paper, markers, crayons, and paint.

△ Let children make their own "grocery list" while adults make their list.

▲ Provide outdoor writing-related activities:

△ Let children draw with sidewalk chalk, paint sidewalks with water, and draw or finger paint on paper.

▲ Incorporate writing-related activities at school:

△ Take advantage of opportunities for writing and drawing that exist within many different school routines and activities.

◼ FOCUSED STRATEGIES

These strategies are for teaching SOME children who are struggling with a component of a skill or whose development is stalled and who need extra help to catch up or keep up. The strategies include a variety of minor adaptations or modifications to daily routines, activities, and environments to meet targeted outcomes at home and in classrooms.

▲ Offer repetitive opportunities for writing across multiple settings with a variety of media.

▲ Let children choose the medium and setting of the writing activity to enhance participation (offer a choice between a dot marker or paint, and let the child indicate their preference by reaching, signing, or vocalizing).

▲ Vary the environments where writing occurs, choosing venues where young children are sitting or standing, active, and alert.

▲ Pay close attention for times when infants are comfortable, alert, and ready to learn, and take advantage of them.

▲ Provide many opportunities for children to watch and observe before they interact with new materials, because some children take a while to warm up to new materials and may need time.

▲ Expand children's repertoire with various writing media once they seem to anticipate what to do and are engaged with a particular medium (once a child has become comfortable using a paintbrush to make scribbles, offer and encourage them to use a marker).

▲ Keep materials and activities short and simple for children who become easily overwhelmed and overstimulated.

▲ Let children set the pace by interacting with materials only as long as they want to do so.

▲ Teach children who cannot speak to use simple signs (MORE, ALL DONE) so they can communicate their preferences.

▲ Learn to recognize children's cues and preferences.

▲ Pair sign language with spoken words for children who are nonverbal or who have hearing impairments.

■ SPECIALIZED STRATEGIES

These strategies for teaching the FEW children who need intensive supports include a variety of specialized, individualized, precise evidence-based strategies to meet children's unique goals/outcomes:

▲ Provide hand-over-hand assistance to demonstrate how to use a writing medium—for example, if using most-to-least prompts:

△ Decrease the amount of hand-over-hand support gradually.

△ Change the location of support to the wrist and then to the forearm before removing physical support altogether.

▲ For children who have motor needs (such as a young child who has cerebral palsy and fisted hands),

△ Use a hook-and-loop or elastic brace to help children grasp writing implements.

△ Add grippers to markers, crayons, and paintbrushes so that they are easier to grasp.

△ Tape several markers or crayons together to make them easier to grasp (also enhances the activity by allowing the child to use several colors at one time).

AEPS-3 Curriculum Resources (Appendix A)

Appendix A in this volume contains numerous additional resources to supplement the AEPS-3 Curriculum. The first part of the appendix presents a list of general curriculum resources, and the second part provides lists of supplementary resources for each individual routine and activity.

AEPS-3 Skills Matrix (Appendix B)

The AEPS-3 Skills Matrix in Appendix B of this volume spotlights individual skills by showing functional application across all routines and activities. Each skills matrix (there are eight total, one for each of the test's eight developmental areas) allows you to select individual AEPS-3 items for children who require an intensive focus on a few skills across routines and activities. For children who have difficulty learning new skills at the level of individual AEPS-3 items, the Foundation Steps (FS) provide an even more granular breakdown of component subskills that are either a sequence of developmental precursors or steps in task analyses.

References

American Academy of Pediatrics. (2016). Media and young minds. *Pediatrics, 138*(5), e20162591. https://doi.org/10.1542/peds.2016-2591

Bronfenbrenner, U. (1994). Ecological models of human development. In *International Encyclopedia of Education, Vol. 3* (2nd ed). Elsevier.

Carta, J. J., & Miller Young, R. (Eds). (2019). *Multi-tiered systems of support for young children: Driving change in early education.* Brookes Publishing Co.

Coleman, M. R., Buysse, V., & Neitzel, J. (2006). *Recognition and Response: An early intervening system for young children at-risk for learning disabilities. Executive summary.* University of North Carolina at Chapel Hill, FPG Child Development Institute.

Collins, B. C. (2022). *Systematic instruction for students with moderate and severe disabilities* (2nd ed.). Brookes Publishing Co.

Cook, B., & Odom, S. L. (2013). Evidence-based practices and implementation science in special education. *Exceptional Children, 79*(3), 135–144.

Copple, C., & Bredekamp, S. (2009). *Developmentally appropriate practice in early childhood programs serving children from birth through age 8* (3rd ed.). National Association for the Education of Young Children.

DEC/NAEYC. (2009). *Early childhood inclusion: A joint position statement of the Division for Early Childhood (DEC) and the National Association for the Education of Young Children (NAEYC).* http://www.dec-sped.org/papers

Division for Early Childhood. (2014). *DEC recommended practices in early intervention/early childhood special education 2014.* Retrieved from https://www.dec-sped.org/dec-recommended-practices

Grisham-Brown, J., & Hemmeter, M. L. (2017). *Blended practices for teaching young children in inclusive settings* (2nd ed.). Brookes Publishing Co.

Harms, T., Cryer, D., & Clifford, R. (2006). *Infant/Toddler Environment Rating Scale–Revised Edition (ITERS-R).* Teachers College Press.

Hemmeter, M. L., Snyder, P. A., Fox, L., & Algina, J. (2016). Evaluating the implementation of the Pyramid Model for promoting social emotional competence in early childhood classrooms. *Topics in Early Childhood Special Education, 36*(3), 133–146.

Johnson, J., Rahn, N., & Bricker, D. (2015). *An activity-based approach to early intervention* (4th ed.). Brookes Publishing Co.

Piaget, J. (1955). *The language and thought of the child.* Meridian Books.

Sandall, S. R., Schwartz, I. S., Joseph, G. E., & Gauvreau, A. (2019). *Building blocks for teaching preschoolers with special needs* (3rd ed.). Brookes Publishing Co.

Skinner, B. F. (1953). *Science and human behavior.* Macmillan.

Children's Book Listed

Christelow, E. (2012). *Five little monkeys jumping in the bath.* Houghton Mifflin Harcourt.

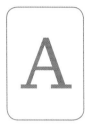

Resources for AEPS®-3 Curriculum Routines and Activities

General Resources

Books

Barton, E. E., & Smith, B. J. (2015). *The preschool inclusion toolbox: How to build and lead a high-quality program.* Brookes Publishing Co.

Bower, E., & Finnie, N. R. (2009). *Finnie's handling the young child with cerebral palsy at home.* Butterworth-Heinemann.

Chen, D. (2008). *Early intervention in action.* Brookes Publishing Co.

Crawford, M., & Weber, B. (2013). *Early intervention every day! Embedding activities in daily routines for young children and their families.* Brookes Publishing Co.

Deiner, P. L. (2008). *Infants & toddlers: Development and curriculum planning* (2nd ed.). Cengage Learning.

Derman-Sparks, L., & Edwards, J. O. (2010). *Anti-bias education for young children and ourselves.* National Association for the Education of Young Children.

Ensher, G., & Clark, D. (2016). *The early years: Foundations for best practice with special children and their families.* ZERO TO THREE.

Grisham-Brown, J., & Hemmeter, M. L. (2017). *Blended practices for teaching young children in inclusive settings* (2nd ed.). Brookes Publishing Co.

Horn, E., Palmer, S. B., Butera, G. D., & Lieber, J. (2016). *Six steps to inclusive preschool curriculum: A UDL-based framework for children's school success.* Brookes Publishing Co.

Johnson, J., Rahn, N., & Bricker, D. (2015). *An activity-based approach to early intervention* (4th ed.). Brookes Publishing Co.

McWilliam, R. A., & Casey, A. M. (2008). *Engagement of every child in the preschool classroom.* Brookes Publishing Co.

Noonan, M. J., & McCormick, L. (2013). *Teaching young children with disabilities in natural environments* (2nd ed.). Brookes Publishing Co.

Richardson-Gibbs, A. M., & Klein, M. D. (2014). *Making preschool inclusion work: Strategies for supporting children, teachers, and programs.* Brookes Publishing Co.

Sandall, S., Schwartz, I., Joseph, G., & Gauvreau, A. (2019). *Building blocks for teaching preschoolers with special needs* (3rd ed.). Brookes Publishing Co.

Schwartz, I., Ashmun, J., McBride, B., Scott, C., & Sandall, S. (2017). *The DATA model for teaching preschoolers with autism: Blending approaches to meet individual needs.* Brookes Publishing Co.

Wittmer, D. S., & Petersen, S. (2017). *Infant and toddler development and responsive program planning: A relationship-based approach* (4th ed.). Pearson.

Journals

Teaching Young Children.   https://www.naeyc.org/resources/pubs/tyc

Teaching Exceptional Children.   https://journals.sagepub.com/home/tcx

Young Children.   https://www.naeyc.org/resources/pubs/yc

Young Exceptional Children.   https://journals.sagepub.com/home/yec

Web Sites

American Printing House for the Blind. https://www.aph.org

Discovery Education. https://www.discoveryeducation.com

Division for Early Childhood. https://www.dec-sped.org

Early Childhood Technical Assistance Center. https://ectacenter.org

National Association for the Education of Young Children. https://www.naeyc.org

Parents. http://www.parents.com

PBS Kids/PBS Learning Media. https://pbskids.org

Positive Parenting Connection. https://www.positiveparentingconnection.net

Results Matter Video Library. https://www.cde.state.co.us/resultsmatter/rmvideoseries

Starfall Education. https://www.starfall.com/h

The STEM Innovation for Inclusion in Early Education Center (STEMI²E²). https://stemie.fpg.unc.edu

ZERO TO THREE. https://www.zerotothree.org

Resources for Individual Routines and Activities

Active & Outdoor Play

Articles and Readings

Early Childhood Today Editorial Staff. (n.d.). Infants & toddlers/activities: Exploring the great outdoors! *Early Childhood Today.* https://www.scholastic.com/teachers/articles/teaching-content/infants -toddlers-activities-exploring-great-outdoors

Gartrell, D., & Sonsteng, K. (2008). Guidance matters: Promote physical activity—It's proactive guidance. *Young Children, 63*(2). https://drjuliejg.files.wordpress.com/2015/02/14-mar-08-yc-gm-phys -activity5.pdf

Honig, A. S. (n.d.). Infants & toddlers: Activities that support outdoor explorations. *Early Childhood Today.* https://www.scholastic.com/teachers/articles/teaching-content/infants-toddlers-activities -support-outdoor-explorations-0

Honig, A. S. (n.d.). Infants and toddlers: Let's go outside! *Early Childhood Today.* https://www.scholastic .com/teachers/articles/teaching-content/infants-toddlers-lets-go-outside

Honig, A. S. (n.d.). Outdoor summer activities for young children. *Early Childhood Today.* https://www .scholastic.com/teachers/articles/teaching-content/outdoor-summer-activities-young-children

Rivkin, M. S. (2001). Problem solving through outdoor play. *Early Childhood Today, 15*(7), 36-43.

Books

Bilton, H. (2010). *Outdoor learning in the early years: Management and innovation* (3rd ed.). Routledge.

Honig, A. S. (2015). *Experiencing nature with young children: Awakening delight, curiosity, and a sense of stewardship.* National Association for the Education of Young Children.

Nelson, E. M. (2012). *Cultivating outdoor classrooms: Designing and implementing child-centered learning environments.* Redleaf Press.

Rivkin, M. S., & Schein, D. (2014). *The great outdoors: Advocating for natural spaces for young children.* National Association for the Education of Young Children.

Sanders, S. (2002). *Active for life: Developmentally appropriate movement programs for young children.* Human Kinetics.

White, J. (2019). *Playing and learning outdoors: The practical guide and sourcebook for excellence in outdoor provision and practice with young children* (3rd ed.). Routledge.

Activities and Ideas to Try

B-Inspired Mama. (n.d.). Outdoor play ideas for kids. *Pinterest.* https://www.pinterest.com /binspiredmama/outdoor-play-ideas-for-kids

Bright Horizons. (n.d.). *17 Fun, low-cost outdoor activities for kids.* https://www.brighthorizons.com /family-resources/fun-outdoor-activities-families

Efe, B. (2015, April 18). 25 Ideas to make outdoor play fun. *Kids Activities Blog.* https://kidsactivitiesblog .com/65939/25-ideas-make-outdoor-play-fun

Cooper, S. (2018, July 3). 44 Preschool outdoor learning ideas. *Teaching 2 and 3 Year Olds.* https:// teaching2and3yearolds.com/44-preschool-outdoor-learning-ideas

Gayle's Preschool Rainbow. (n.d.). *Outdoor play.* http://www.preschoolrainbow.org/preschool -outdoor.htm

Learning 4 Kids. (n.d.). *Active play.* https://www.learning4kids.net/category/active-play

McLennan, D. P. (2017). Math learning—and a touch of science—in the outdoor world. *Teaching Young Children, 10*(4). https://www.naeyc.org/resources/pubs/tyc/apr2017/math-learning-outdoors

No Time for Flash Cards. (2012, March 7). *50 Simple outdoor activities for kids.* https://www.notimeforflashcards.com/2012/03/50-simple-outdoor-activities-for-kids.html

Virtual Lab School. (n.d.). *Infants & toddlers learning environments—The outdoor environment: Designing for engagement.* https://www.virtuallabschool.org/infants-toddlers/learning-environments/lesson-3?module=4151

Virtual Lab School. (n.d.). *Preschool learning environments—The outdoor environment: Designing for learning.* https://www.virtuallabschool.org/preschool/learning-environments/lesson-3?module=3601

Virtual Lab School. (n.d.). *Preschool physical development—Supporting physical development: Outdoor environments and experiences.* https://www.virtuallabschool.org/preschool/physical-development/lesson-4?module=7541

Virtual Lab School. (n.d.). *School-age learning environments—The outdoor environment: Designing for learning.* https://www.virtuallabschool.org/school-age/learning-environments/lesson-3

Videos

McDaniel, L. (2014, August 17). *Video model of outside play* [Video]. YouTube. https://www.youtube.com/watch?v=PbcVe7fDu94

STARNET: Early Childhood. (2016, May 9). *Engaging young children in the outdoor environment* [Video]. YouTube. https://www.youtube.com/watch?v=FrEfhE5VuSQ

Arrival & Departure

Articles and Readings

Tours, S. B., & Dennis, L. R. (2015). Easing first day jitters: Strategies for successful home-to-school transitions. *Young Children, 70*(4): 84–89. https://www.naeyc.org/resources/pubs/yc/sep2015/easing-first-day-jitters

Activities and Ideas to Try

Autism Classroom Resources. (n.d.). Creating learning opportunities during arrival and departure. https://autismclassroomresources.com/5-incidental-teaching-opportunities-during-arrival-departure

Head Start Early Learning and Knowledge Center. (n.d.). *Supporting transitions: Resources for building collaboration.* https://eclkc.ohs.acf.hhs.gov/transitions/article/supporting-transitions-resources-building-collaboration

National Association for the Education of Young Children. (n.d.). *Routines and transitions.* https://www.naeyc.org/resources/topics/routines-and-transitions

Not Just Cute with Amanda Morgan. (2009, August 24). *Terrific transitions at preschool arrival and departure.* https://notjustcute.com/2009/08/24/terrific-transitions-at-preschool-arrival-and-departure

Preschool Plan-It. (n.d.). *5 Transition activities + tips for your preschool classroom.* https://www.preschool-plan-it.com/transition-activities.html

Videos

McDaniel, Lindy. *Goodbye ritual for a pre-K classroom* [Video]. YouTube:

- Option #1 (2014, September 1): https://www.youtube.com/watch?v=_8aZRPgK3yg
- Option #2 (2014, September 13): https://www.youtube.com/watch?v=jPAnZwEvJuk
- Option #3 (n.d.): https://www.youtube.com/watch?v=KaCsaYUA5PI
- Option #4 (n.d.): https://www.youtube.com/watch?v=f3m0h-Kgajw

McDaniel, Lindy. (n.d.). *Our ECSE classroom's schedule: Part one—Arrival & daily jobs* [Video]. YouTube. https://www.youtube.com/watch?v=uwFA7llHqXk

Seeing is Believing. (2012, February 9). *Arrival routines in action* [Video]. YouTube. https://www.youtube.com/watch?v=UlQQRVso4d8

Art

Articles and Readings

Bernstein, P. (2013). Why art and creativity are important. *Parents.* https://www.parents.com /toddlers-preschoolers/development/intellectual/why-art-and-creativity-are-important

Bongiorno, L. (2014). How process-focused art experiences support preschoolers. *Teaching Young Children, 7*(3). https://www.naeyc.org/resources/pubs/tyc/feb2014/process-art-experiences

PBS Kids for Parents. (n.d.). *Create Art!* https://www.pbs.org/parents/art

Books

Editors of Teaching Young Children. (2015). *Expressing creativity in preschool.* National Association for the Education of Young Children.

Koralek, D. (2005). *Spotlight on young children and the creative arts.* National Association for the Education of Young Children.

Activities and Ideas to Try

The Artful Parent. (n.d.). *500+ Kids arts and crafts activities.* https://artfulparent.com/kids-arts -crafts-activities-500-fun-artful-things-kids

Early Learning Ideas. (n.d.). *Art and crafts.* https://earlylearningideas.com/category/art-crafts

Education.com. (n.d.). *Preschool arts & crafts activities.* https://www.education.com/activity/preschool /arts-and-crafts

Gryphon House. (n.d.). *Free art activities for all ages.* https://www.gryphonhouse.com/activities/category /post-art

Hands On As We Grow. (n.d.). *What toddler crafts and art projects can we do? 30 Ideas.* https:// handsonaswegrow.com/30-creative-toddler-craft-art-projects

JumpStart. (n.d.). *Art activities.* https://www.jumpstart.com/parents/activities/art-activities

Learning 4 Kids. (n.d.). *Craft.* https://www.learning4kids.net/category/craft

PBS Kids for Parents. (n.d.). *Arts.* https://www.pbs.org/parents/learn-grow/all-ages/arts

Play to Learn Preschool. (n.d.). *Art projects.* https://playtolearnpreschool.us/art

Preschool Learning Online. (n.d.). *PreK art activities, easy kids crafts & painting ideas.* https://www .preschoollearningonline.com/preschool-art.html

Teaching 2 and 3 Year Olds. (n.d.). *Archives: Art.* https://teaching2and3yearolds.com/category/art

Van't Hul, J. (2015, November 6). 7 Simple art activities for toddlers. *The Artful Parent.* https://artfulparent. com/7-simple-art-activities-for-toddlers

Videos

5-Minutes Crafts PLAY. (2018, February 10). *17 Educational crafts for preschoolers* [Video]. YouTube. https://www.youtube.com/watch?v=6CwFlhHZ97A

5-Minutes Crafts PLAY. (2018, October 5). *17 Fun educational crafts for toddlers* [Video]. YouTube. https://www.youtube.com/watch?v=FwdzRYbBh00

5-Minutes Crafts PLAY. (2019, June 17). *16 Creative drawing hacks for kids* [Video]. YouTube. https://www.youtube.com/watch?v=xSsdnC896pU

Clubbhouse Kids. (2017, May 14). *Ideas for art in the infant/toddler classroom* [Video]. YouTube. https://www.youtube.com/watch?v=X9F63Q6wcaQ

Preschool Learning Online. (n.d.). *Preschool kids art ideas: Pre K art activities* [Video]. YouTube. https://www.youtube.com/watch?v=9Y4HIiWMnGs

Bath Time

Activities and Ideas to Try

Alyssa. (n.d.). 18 Bath activities for kids. *Realistic Mama.* https://www.therealisticmama.com/bath-activities-for-kids

Braley, P. (2014, May 2). 10 Fun bath time activities for kids. *The Inspired Treehouse.* https://theinspiredtreehouse.com/?s=10+fun+bath

Block Play

Articles and Readings

Anderson, C. (2010). Blocks: A versatile learning tool for yesterday, today, and tomorrow. *Young Children, 65*(2).

Block building and make-believe for every child. (2010). *Teaching Young Children, 3*(3).

Blocks: Great learning tools from infancy through the primary grades. (2015). *Young Children, 70*(1). https://www.naeyc.org/resources/pubs/yc/mar2015

Kuder, B. N., & Hojnoski, R. L. (2016). Under construction: Strategic changes in the block area to promote engagement and learning. *Young Exceptional Children, 21*(2), 76–91. https://doi.org/10.1177/1096250616649224

Wise Lindeman, K., & McKendry Anderson, E. (2016). Does your block center promote 21st century skills? A checklist for teachers. *Teaching Young Children, 9*(3). https://www.naeyc.org/resources/pubs/tyc/feb2016/does-your-block-center-promote-21st-century

Books

Chalufour, I., & Worth, K. (2004). *Building structures with young children.* Redleaf Press.

Activities and Ideas to Try

Fun Learning for Kids. (n.d.). *7 Toddler learning activities with Mega Bloks.* https://funlearningforkids.com/7-toddler-learning-activities-with-mega-bloks

Hands On As We Grow. (n.d.). 47 Super fun block activities for preschoolers. *Pinterest.* https://www.pinterest.com/pin/283586107761540617

Hands On As We Grow. (n.d.). *Blocks of fun! 47 Block activities for preschoolers.* https://handsonaswegrow.com/lots-of-blocks-activities

Levin, V. (n.d.). Blocks center set up in preschool. *Pre-K Pages.* https://www.pre-kpages.com/blocks_center

Stephens, K. (2007). Block play activities for home, child care, or school. *Parenting Exchange.* https://www.easternflorida.edu/community-resources/child-development-centers/parent-resource-library/documents/block-play-activities.pdf

Teaching 2 and 3 Year Olds. (n.d.). *Archives: Blocks.* https://teaching2and3yearolds.com/category/blocks

Circle Time

Activities and Ideas to Try

Barton, E. E., Reichow, B., Wolery, M., & Chen, C.-I. (2011). We can all participate! Adapting circle time for children with autism. *Young Exceptional Children, 14*(2): 2–21. https://doi.org/10.1177/1096250610393681

Cooper, S. (2013, September 1). Circle time activities. *Teaching 2 and 3 Year Olds.* https://teaching2and3yearolds.com/circle-time-activities

FlannelBoardFun. (n.d.). Circle time activities. *Pinterest.* https://www.pinterest.com/FlannelBoardFun/circle-time-activities

Gayle's Preschool Rainbow. Preschool large group and circle activities. http://www.preschoolrainbow.org/activities-large.htm

Laura. (2011, February 15). Making circle time successful. *Teach Me to Talk!* https://teachmetotalk .com/2011/02/15/making-circle-time-successful

Levin, V. (n.d.). Circle time tips for preschool and pre-K teachers. *Pre-K Pages.* https://www.pre-kpages .com/circle_time

Luckenbill, J. (2011). Circle time puppets: Teaching social skills. *Teaching Young Children, 4*(4). https:// www.yumpu.com/en/document/read/4736782/circle-time-puppets-teaching-social-skills

Play to Learn Preschool. (n.d.). Circle time. https://playtolearnpreschool.us/category/circle-time

Teaching 2 and 3 Year Olds. (n.d.). *Archives: Circle time.* https://teaching2and3yearolds.com/category /circle-time

Videos

McDaniel, L. (n.d.). *Another way to set up large group in pre-K classrooms* [Video]. YouTube. https://www .youtube.com/watch?v=5rKsLZge8GI

McDaniel, L. (n.d.). *How to have successful large group sessions* [Video]. YouTube. https://www.youtube .com/watch?v=5svHUqvsCgI

Preschool Learning Online. (n.d.). *Preschool circle time songs, how to start circle time with a song, ideas, activities pre K* [Video]. YouTube. https://www.youtube.com/watch?v=6iWwLTS8IDI

Diapering, Toileting, & Handwashing

Articles and Readings

Suppo, J. L., & Mayton, M. R. (2012). A portable potty plan for children with autism. *Young Exceptional Children, 15*(4). https://doi.org/10.1177/1096250612451758

Books

Brucks, B. (2016). *Potty training in 3 days: The step-by-step plan for a clean break from dirty diapers.* Althea Publishers.

Capucilli, A. S. (2000). *The potty book for boys.* Barron's Educational Series.

Capucilli, A. S. (2000). *The potty book for girls.* Barron's Educational Series.

Patricelli, L. (2010). *Potty.* Candlewick Press.

Activities and Ideas to Try

Beck, C. (2016). Tips for how to teach kids potty training. *The OT Toolbox.* https://www.theottoolbox.com /tips-for-how-to-teach-kids-potty

Child Care Aware of North Dakota. (n.d.). *Diapering time activities.* https://www.ndchildcare.org/file _download/d84e8254-f9f7-41fe-b035-a30e8920d894

Child Care Aware of North Dakota. (n.d.). *Toilet (potty) training checklist.* https://ndchildcareorg .presencehost.net/file_download/a6ac918e-4075-4137-9dc1-6eac9df0493c

Parents. (n.d.). *Diapering.* https://www.parents.com/baby/diapers

Poole, C. (n.d.). Infants and toddlers/communication with families: How to create diapering and toileting routines. *Scholastic.* https://www.scholastic.com/teachers/articles/teaching-content/infants -toddlerscommunication-families-how-create-diapering-and-toileting-routines

Virtual Lab School. (n.d.). Staying healthy: Diapering and toileting. https://www.virtuallabschool.org /fcc/healthy-environments/lesson-3

Videos

Child Care Aware ND. (2017, December 18). Diapering [Video]. YouTube. https://www.youtube.com /playlist?list=PLsqrHdiqnOiuRgDvTLnxYRkyR9hUuvQOq

PBS Learning Media. (n.d.). *Hand washing* [Video]. https://www.pbslearningmedia.org/resource /eb12ac7a-a6fe-4758-80e2-7b12f588beba/hand-washing/#.WTtvq2grLIU

PBS Learning Media. (n.d.). *Prince Wednesday goes potty: Daniel Tiger's neighborhood* [Video]. https://www.pbslearningmedia.org/resource/36e64535-03e7-48cf-9d85-a7b890cb9938/prince -wednesday-goes-potty-daniel-tigers-neighborhood/#.WTtyk2jyvIU

PBS Learning Media. (n.d.). *When you have to go potty, stop and go right away! Daniel Tiger's neighborhood* [Video]. https://www.pbslearningmedia.org/resource/b6e14698-8253-44b6-acde-9c39b5d8280d/when-you-have-to-go-potty-stop-and-go-right-away-daniel-tigers-neighborhood/#.WTtyMmjyvIU

Virtual Lab School. (n.d.). *Stay healthy: Diapering and toileting* (infants and toddlers):
- *Helping children after accidents* [Video] (https://stream.virtuallabschool.org/healthy/3915/3915-480.mp4)
- *Diapering correctly with sensitive interactions* [Video] (https://stream.virtuallabschool.org/healthy/5349/5349-480.mp4)
- *Changing diapers supports development* [Video] (https://stream.virtuallabschool.org/healthy/3743/3743-480.mp4)

Virtual Lab School. (n.d.). *Stay healthy: Diapering and toileting* (preschool):
- *Restroom hygiene* [Video] (https://stream.virtuallabschool.org/healthy/3860/3860-480.mp4)
- *Helping children after accidents* [Video] (https://stream.virtuallabschool.org/healthy/3866/3866-480.mp4)

Dramatic Play

Articles and Readings

Barton, E. E., & Pavilanis, R. (2012). Teaching pretend play to young children with autism. *Young Exceptional Children, 15*(1). https://doi.org/10.1177/1096250611424106?journalCode=yeca

Bright Horizons Education Team. *The importance of pretend play in child development.* https://www.brighthorizons.com/family-resources/importance-of-pretend-play-in-child-development

Early Learning Ideas. (n.d.). This is what you need to know about dramatic play. https://earlylearningideas.com/dramatic-play

McEntire, N. (2009). Pretend play in the early childhood classroom. *Childhood Education, 85*(3).

Books

Editors of Teaching Young Children. (2015). *Expressing creativity in preschool.* National Association for the Education of Young Children.

Koralek, D. (2005). *Spotlight on young children and the creative arts.* National Association for the Education of Young Children.

Activities and Ideas to Try

Dramatic play—Every day. (2005). *Texas Child Care.* https://www.childcarequarterly.com/winter05_story2a.html

Illinois Early Learning Project. (n.d.). *Drama and young children.* https://illinoisearlylearning.org/tipsheets/drama

Learning 4 Kids. (n.d.). *Pretend.* https://www.learning4kids.net/category/pretend

Levin, V. (n.d.). Dramatic play. *Pre-K Pages.* https://www.pre-kpages.com/category/dramatic-play

PennState Extension. (n.d.). Dramatic play: Let's think beyond the housekeeping corner! https://extension.psu.edu/programs/betterkidcare/knowledge-areas/environment-curriculum/activities/all-activities/dramatic-play-beyond-housekeeping-corner

Play to Learn Preschool. (n.d.). *Dramatic play.* https://playtolearnpreschool.us/dramatic-play

Preschool Learning Online. (n.d.). *Dramatic play preschool ideas & activities for children in preschool.* https://www.preschoollearningonline.com/dramatic-play.html

Teaching 2 and 3 Year Olds. (n.d.). *Archives: Dramatic play.* https://teaching2and3yearolds.com/category/dramatic-play

Videos

McDaniel, L. (n.d.). *Pretend play center in an early childhood classroom* [Video]. YouTube. https://www.youtube.com/watch?v=oh2agWaSSkU

Dressing

Activities and Ideas to Try

Beck, C. (2016, June 24). Functional skills for kids. *The OT Toolbox.* https://www.theottoolbox.com/functional-skills-for-kids

Brill, A. (2012, June 13). Giant list of self-care skills for babies, toddlers, and preschoolers. *Positive Parenting Connection.* https://www.positiveparentingconnection.net/giant-list-of-self-care-skills-for-babiestoddlers-and-preschoolers

Family Connect for Parents of Children with Visual Impairments. (n.d.). Teaching bathing and dressing skills for dual diagnosis children. https://familyconnect.org/multiple-disabilities/independent-living-skills/bathing-and-dressing/135

Videos

The Kids' Picture Show. (2013, April 22). *Getting dressed: How to put on a T-shirt* [Video]. YouTube. https://www.youtube.com/watch?v=WWNlgvtYcEs

The Kids' Picture Show. (2013, July 4). *Getting dressed: How to put on pants* [Video]. YouTube. https://www.youtube.com/watch?v=oMae4XZnxTw

Field Trips

Articles and Readings

National Association for the Education of Young Children. (2013). Get to know the NEW children's librarian. *Teaching Young Children, 7*(2), 28.

National Association for the Education of Young Children. (2016). Family field trips: Museums. *Teaching Young Children, 9*(4). https://www.naeyc.org/resources/pubs/tyc/apr2016/backpack/family-field-trips-museums

Resources for incorporating books throughout the curriculum. (2007). *Young Children, 62*(3).

Books

Abbot, E. A. (2020). *Family field trip: Explore art, food, music, and nature with kids.* Chronicle Books.

Brown, M. (2003). *D.W.'s library card.* Scholastic.

Buhr, E. (2018). *Little walks, big adventures: 50+ ideas for exploring with toddlers.* Gryphon House.

Cousins, L. (2013). *Maisy goes to the museum.* Candlewick.

Feldman, T. (2018). *Let's go to our zoo (Smithsonian Kids).* Cottage Door Press.

Hill, E. (1996). *Spot goes to the park.* Puffin.

Jalongo, M. R. (2004). *Young children and picture books* (2nd ed.). National Association for the Education of Young Children.

McAnulty, S. (2018). *Max explains everything: Grocery store expert.* G.P. Putnam Sons.

Parish, H. (2013). *Amelia Bedelia's first field trip.* Greenwillow Books.

Parish, H., & Swear, L. (2005). *Amelia Bedelia, Bookworm.* Greenwillow Books.

Activities and Ideas to Try

Colorín Colorado. *Your library.* https://www.colorincolorado.org/your-library

Crouch, M. (2016, January 5). 4 Field trips that are perfect for preschoolers. *Parents.* https://www.parents.com/toddlers-preschoolers/activities/4-field-trips-that-are-perfect-for-preschoolers

Illinois Early Learning Project. (n.d.). *Outdoor field trips with preschoolers: Preparing with the children.* https://illinoisearlylearning.org/tipsheets/field-preparing

ilovelibraries. *For parents.* http://www.ilovelibraries.org/parents

Kiehl, K. L. (2016). Inspired by museums—Both outside and inside the classroom. *Teaching Young Children, 9*(4). https://www.naeyc.org/resources/pubs/tyc/apr2016/inspired-museums-outside-and-inside-classroom

Levin, V. (n.d.). Field trip ideas for preschool and kindergarten. *Pre-K Pages.* https://www.pre-kpages.com/field-trips

Levin, V. (n.d.). Preschool classroom library center. *Pre-K Pages.* https://www.pre-kpages.com/classlibrary

Not Just Cute with Amanda Morgan. (2010, August 16). Why don't you teach reading? A look at emergent literacy (series). https://notjustcute.com/2010/08/16/why-dont-you-teach-reading-a-look-at-emergent-literacy

SAG-AFTRA Foundation. (n.d.). *Storyline online.* https://www.storylineonline.net/library

Simply Daycare. (n.d.). *Field trip ideas.* https://www.simplydaycare.com/field-trip-ideas.html

U.S. Department of Education. *Helping your child use the library.* https://www2.ed.gov/pubs/parents/Library/Interested.html

Videos

Home Grown Books. (n.d.). *Resources* [series of videos for emergent readers]. https://homegrownbooksnyc.com/videos

South Florida PBS. (n.d.). Take a field trip [YouTube series]. https://www.youtube.com/c/WPBT2/search?query=kidvision

ZERO TO THREE. (2016, February 2). *Babies, toddlers, and early reading* [Video]. YouTube. https://www.zerotothree.org/resources/20-babies-toddlers-and-early-reading

Math

Articles and Readings

Burton, M. (2010). Five strategies for creating meaningful mathematics experiences in the primary years. *Young Children, 65*(6). https://www.researchgate.net/publication/285756551_Five_strategies_for_creating_meaningful_mathematics_experiences_in_the_primary_years

Geist, K., & Geist, E. (2008). Do re mi, 1-2-3 that's how easy math can be: Using music to support emergent mathematics. *Young Children, 63*(2). https://www.researchgate.net/publication/290004564_Do_re_mi_1-2-3_that%27s_how_easy_math_can_be_Using_music_to_support_emergent_mathematics

Moomaw, S., & Davis, J. A. (2010). STEM comes to preschool. *Young Children, 65*(5). https://www.researchgate.net/publication/292035679_STEM_comes_to_preschool

National Association for the Education of Young Children & National Council of Teachers of Mathematics. (2010). *Early childhood mathematics: Promoting good beginnings* [Position statement]. https://www.naeyc.org/sites/default/files/globally-shared/downloads/PDFs/resources/position-statements/psmath.pdf

National Association for the Education of Young Children. (2017). *Teaching Young Children, 11*(1). [October/November 2017 issue focused on math.]

Notari-Syverson, A., & Sadler, F. H. (2008). Math is for everyone: Strategies for supporting early mathematical competencies in young children. *Young Exceptional Children, 11*(3). https://www.researchgate.net/publication/240731670_Math_Is_for_Everyone_Strategies_for_Supporting_Early_Mathematical_Competencies_in_Young_Children

Pecaski McLennan, D. (2014). Making math meaningful for young children. *Teaching Young Children, 8*(1). https://www.naeyc.org/resources/pubs/tyc/oct2014/making-math-meaningful

Rosen, D., & Hoffman, J. (2009). Integrating concrete and virtual manipulatives in early childhood mathematics. *Young Children, 64*(3). https://www.researchgate.net/publication/287695795_Integrating_concrete_and_virtual_manipulatives_in_early_childhood_mathematics

Books

Copley, J. V. (2003). *Showcasing mathematics for the young child: Activities for three-, four-, and five-year-olds.* National Association for the Education of Young Children.

Copley, J. V. (2010). *The young child and mathematics.* National Association for the Education of Young Children.

Counsell, S., Escalada, L., Geiken, R., Sander, M., Uhlenberg, J., Meeteren, B. V., Yoshizawa, S., & Zan, B. (2016). *STEM learning with young children: Inquiry teaching with ramps and pathways.* National Association for the Education of Young Children.

Early Math Collaborative. (2013). *Big ideas of early mathematics: What teachers of young children need to know.* Pearson.

Editors of Teaching Young Children. (2015). *Exploring math and science in preschool.* National Association for the Education of Young Children.

Heroman, C. (2017). *Making and tinkering with STEM: Solving design challenges with young children.* National Association for the Education of Young Children.

Kotsopoulos, D., & Lee, J. (2014). *Let's talk about math: The LittleCounters approach to building early math skills.* Brookes Publishing Co.

Krogh, S., & Slentz, K. (2001). *The early childhood curriculum: Inquiry learning through integration.* Erlbaum.

Moomaw, S. (2011). *Teaching mathematics in early childhood.* Brookes Publishing Co.

Shillady, A. (2016). *Spotlight on young children: Exploring math.* National Association for the Education of Young Children.

Activities and Ideas to Try

Arkansas Child Development and Early Learning Standards. (2018). Mathematical thinking. In *Strategies and activities: Infant toddler.* https://ecep.uark.edu/_resources/pdf_other/06_division_materials/strategies_activities_infant_toddler2018.pdf

Cooper, S. (2020, March 6). The ultimate collection of preschool math activities. *Teaching 2 and 3 Year Olds.* https://teaching2and3yearolds.com/the-ultimate-collection-preschool-math-activities

Education.com. (n.d.). *Preschool math activities.* https://www.education.com/activity/preschool/math

Education.com. (n.d.). *Preschool math games.* https://www.education.com/games/preschool/math

Hanke, H. (n.d.). Fun activities to promote math skills. *BabyCenter.* https://www.babycenter.com/0_fun-activities-to-promote-math-skills_64460.bc

Institute of Education Sciences. (2014). *Educator's practice guide: Teaching math to young children.* What Works Clearinghouse. https://ies.ed.gov/ncee/wwc/Docs/PracticeGuide/early_math_pg_111313.pdf

JumpStart. (n.d.). *Math activities for kids.* https://www.jumpstart.com/parents/activities/math-activities

Learning 4 Kids. (n.d.). *Play categories: Numbers.* https://www.learning4kids.net/category/numbers

Levin, V. (n.d.). Math activities. *Pre-K Pages.* https://www.pre-kpages.com/math

National Association for the Education of Young Children. (n.d.). *Math talk with infants and toddlers.* https://www.naeyc.org/our-work/families/math-talk-infants-and-toddlers

PBS Kids. (n.d.). *Math games.* https://pbskids.org/games/math

PBS Kids for Parents. (n.d.). *Math.* https://www.pbs.org/parents/learn-grow/all-ages/math

Play to Learn Preschool. (n.d.). *Learning center: Math.* https://playtolearnpreschool.us/category/math

Teaching-Tiny-Tots.com. (n.d.). *Toddler math.* http://www.teaching-tiny-tots.com/toddler-math.html

Thayer, A. (n.d.). 15 Hands-on math activities for preschoolers. *Teaching Mama.* https://teachingmama.org/15-hands-on-math-activities-preschoolers

ZERO TO THREE. (n.d.). *Help your child develop early math skills.* https://www.zerotothree.org/resources/299-help-your-child-develop-early-math-skills

Videos

McDaniel, L. (n.d.). *Building a math center in an early childhood special needs classroom* [Video]. YouTube. https://www.youtube.com/watch?v=2i7XO0YJC3Y

PBS Learning Media. (n.d.). *Math resources* [Video series]. https://www.pbslearningmedia.org/math

ZERO TO THREE. (n.d.). Let's talk about math: Early math video series. https://www.zerotothree.org/resources/series/let-s-talk-about-math-early-math-video-series

Meals & Snacks

Articles and Readings

Bruns, D., & Thompson, S. D. (2011). Time to eat: Improving mealtimes of children with autism. *Young Exceptional Children, 14*(4). https://www.researchgate.net/publication/256447157_Time_to_Eat _Improving_Mealtimes_of_Young_Children_With_Autism

Bruns, D., & Thompson, S. D. (2014). Turning mealtimes into learning opportunities: Integrating feeding goals into IEPs. *Teaching Exceptional Children, 46*(6), 179–186. https://doi.org/10.1177 /0040059914534619

Family Connect for Parents of Children with Visual Impairments. (n.d.). Supporting the development of eating skills for children with multiple disabilities. https://familyconnect.org/multiple-disabilities /independent-living-skills/eating-skills

Make mealtimes learning times. (2014). *Teaching Young Children, 7*(5). https://www.naeyc.org/resources /pubs/tyc/jun2014/backpack/make-mealtimes-learning-times

Thompson, S. D., Bruns, D., & Rains, K. W. (2010). Picky eating habits or sensory processing issues? Exploring feeding difficulties in infants and toddlers. *Young Exceptional Children, 13*(2). https://www .researchgate.net/publication/249836360_Picky_Eating_Habits_or_Sensory_Processing_Issues _Exploring_Feeding_Difficulties_in_Infants_and_Toddlers

Books

Bruns, D. A., & Thompson, S. D. (2012). *Feeding challenges in young children.* Brookes Publishing Co.

DK Publishing. (2012). *Baby touch and feel: Mealtime.* DK Children.

Fernando, N., & Potock, M. (2015). *Raising a healthy, happy eater: A parent's handbook: A stage-by-stage guide to setting your child on the path to adventurous eating.* The Experiment, LLC.

Satter, E. (1987). *How to get your kid to eat: But not too much.* Bull Publishing.

Verdick, E., & Heinlen, M. (2011). *Mealtime.* Toddler tools. Free Spirit Publishing.

Activities and Ideas to Try

New York State Department of Health. (2012). *Chatting with children at mealtimes: Creating a climate for communication.* https://www.health.ny.gov/prevention/nutrition/resources/chattingmeal.htm

Parents. (n.d.). *Eating and nutrition.* https://www.parents.com/kids/nutrition

Parents. (n.d.). *Feeding.* https://www.parents.com/baby/feeding

Play to Learn Preschool. (n.d.). *Preschool snack time.* https://playtolearnpreschool.us/preschool-snack -time-2

Virtual Lab School. (n.d.). *Infants & toddlers: Healthy environments | Staying healthy: Nutrition, feeding, and physical activity.* https://www.virtuallabschool.org/infants-toddlers/healthy/lesson-5?module=3446

Virtual Lab School. (n.d.). *Preschool: Healthy environments | Staying healthy: Nutrition and physical activity.* https://www.virtuallabschool.org/preschool/healthy/lesson-5?module=3076

ZERO TO THREE. (2010, February 20). *Creating routines for love and learning.* https://www.zerotothree .org/resources/223-creating-routines-for-love-and-learning

Videos

McDaniel, L. (n.d.). *Preparing for snack time in a pre-K classroom* [Video]. YouTube. https://www.youtube .com/watch?v=ebfVan-Byzc

PBS Learning Media. (n.d.). *Katerina finally tries a new food: Daniel Tiger's neighborhood* [Video]. https:// www.pbslearningmedia.org/resource/4f0c441c-2af8-437d-a102-b9b2c356fcce/katerina-finally -tries-a-new-food/#.WTtzlmgrLIU

PBS Learning Media. (n.d.). *Trying tomatoes: Daniel Tiger's neighborhood* [Video]. https://www.pbslearn ingmedia.org/resource/30c0868b-10fb-4f10-bfd5-31052d594d07/trying-tomatoes/#.WTtzV2grLIU

PBS Learning Media. (n.d.). *Trying veggie spaghetti: Daniel Tiger's neighborhood* [Video]. https://www .pbslearningmedia.org/resource/e3096f63-3d1f-4e16-bb0f-a46ca56e0ee3/trying-veggie -spaghetti/#.WTtwNmjyvIU

WUCF TV. (2018, June 14). *WUCF's Snack Hacks* [Video series]. https://www.wucf.org/learn/pbs-kids /snack-hacks

Music & Movement

Articles and Readings

Cooper, J. (2016). Integrating music, drama, and dance helps children explore and learn. *Teaching Young Children, 9*(4). https://www.naeyc.org/resources/pubs/tyc/apr2016/integrating-music-drama-and-dance-helps-children

National Association for the Education of Young Children. (2010). *Young Children, 65*(2). [March 2010 issue focused on music and other creative arts.]

Orlowski, M. A., & Hart, A. (2010). Go! Including movement during routines and transitions. *Young Children, 65*(5). https://www.researchgate.net/publication/294701367_Go_Movement_during_routines_and_transitions

PBS Kids for Parents. (n.d.). *Make and Play Music!* https://www.pbs.org/parents/music

Books

Editors of Teaching Young Children. (2015). *Expressing creativity in preschool.* National Association for the Education of Young Children.

Kotowicz, A. (2019). *Winter song: A day in the life of a kid.* ArtsKindred.

Koralek, D. (2005). *Spotlight on young children and the creative arts.* National Association for the Education of Young Children.

Activities and Ideas to Try

Arkansas Child Development and Early Learning Standards. (2018). Creativity and aesthetics. In *Strategies and activities: Infant toddler.* https://ecep.uark.edu/_resources/pdf_other/06_division_materials/strategies_activities_infant_toddler2018.pdf

Gryphon House. (2015, October 13). *Music and movement activities for infants, toddlers & preschoolers.* https://www.gryphonhouse.com/activities/music-and-movement-activities-for-infants-toddlers-preschoolers

Honig, A. S. (n.d.). Infants and toddlers/Activities: Musical activities *Scholastic.* https://www.scholastic.com/teachers/articles/teaching-content/infants-toddlersactivities-musical-activities

Illinois Early Learning Project. (n.d.). *Sing, play, and hear: Music's in the air.* https://illinoisearlylearning.org/tipsheets/sing

Kids Environment Kids Health, National Institute of Environmental Health Sciences. (n.d.). *Songs.* https://kids.niehs.nih.gov/games/songs/index.htm

Lerner, C., & Parlakian, R. (2016, August 11). Beyond Twinkle, Twinkle: Using music with infants and toddlers. *ZERO TO THREE.* https://www.zerotothree.org/resources/1514-beyond-twinkle-twinkle-using-music-with-infants-and-toddlers

Levin, V. (n.d.). Music in the classroom. *Pre-K Pages.* https://www.pre-kpages.com/music-in-the-classroom

Preschool Learning Online. *Learning songs for preschoolers.* https://www.preschoollearningonline.com/preschool-songs.html

Teaching 2 and 3 Year Olds. (n.d.). *Music and movement.* https://teaching2and3yearolds.com/category/music-and-movement

Nap & Sleep

Articles and Readings

Mendola, W. (2017). Nap time is for letting go. *Teaching Young Children, 10*(2). https://www.naeyc.org/resources/pubs/tyc/dec2016/nap-time-letting-go?utm_content=buffer8f76e&utm_medium=social&utm_source=facebook.com&utm_campaign=buffer

Pacheco, D. (2020, September 20). Children and sleep. *Sleep Foundation.* https://www.sleepfoundation.org/articles/children-and-sleep

Books

Verdick, E., & Heinlen, M. (2012). *Bedtime.* Toddler tools. Free Spirit Publishing.

Verdick, E., & Heinlen, M. (2011). *Naptime.* Toddler tools. Free Spirit Publishing.

Activities and Ideas to Try

Baby Sleep Site. (n.d.). *Baby and toddler sleep resources for childcare providers.* https://www.babysleepsite .com/childcare-resources

Ben-Joseph, E. P. (n.d.). All about sleep. *KidsHealth.* https://kidshealth.org/en/parents/sleep.html

Cleveland Clinic. (n.d.). *Sleep in toddlers and preschoolers.* https://my.clevelandclinic.org/health /articles/14302-sleep-in-toddlers–preschoolers

Harvey, H. (n.d.). Encouraging healthy sleep habits. *National Association for the Education of Young Children.* https://www.naeyc.org/our-work/families/encouraging-healthy-sleep-habits

Head Start Early Childhood Learning and Knowledge Center. (n.d.). *News you can use: The culture of sleep and child care.* https://eclkc.ohs.acf.hhs.gov/school-readiness/article/news-you-can-use-culture -sleep-child-care

Levin, V. (n.d.). Nap time tips for preschool teachers. *Pre-K Pages.* https://www.pre-kpages.com/nap -time-routine

Norman, R. (n.d.). *How to get your littles to sleep in and take longer naps.* https://amotherfarfromhome .com/help-babies-toddlers-sleep-later

Pantley, E. (n.d.). Eight sleep tips for toddlers & preschoolers. *Child Development Institute.* https:// childdevelopmentinfo.com/ages-stages/toddler-preschooler-development-parenting/sleep-tips -toddlers-preschoolers/#gs.xhuf6w

Parents. (n.d.). *Napping.* https://www.parents.com/kids/sleep/naps

Parents. (n.d.). *Sleep.* https://www.parents.com/kids/sleep

Rachel. (2014, May 2). 16 Nap time play ideas. *Kids Activities Blog.* https://kidsactivitiesblog.com/52377 /16-nap-time-play-ideas

Videos

PBS Learning Media. (n.d.). *The bedtime song: Daniel Tiger's neighborhood* [Video]. https://www.pbslearn ingmedia.org/resource/e4057574-ad19-48f3-811f-52d04f7afffc/the-bedtime-song/#.WTtxyWjyvIU

PBS Learning Media. (n.d.). *Finn's bedtime: Daniel Tiger's neighborhood* [Video]. https://www.pbslearn ingmedia.org/resource/44594303-a357-4b85-9f2b-700b4c45a0ff/finns-bedtime/#.WTtxhGgrLIU

PBS Learning Media. (n.d.). *Storytime: Daniel Tiger's neighborhood* [Video]. https://www.pbslearningme dia.org/resource/2ea5c444-11a9-4a84-b3ab-38c6a1b268c0/storytime/#.WTtxfWgrLIU

Science (Growing and Ready levels only)

Articles and Readings

Head Start Early Childhood Learning and Knowledge Center. (n.d.). *News you can use: Early science learn-ing for infants and toddlers.* https://eclkc.ohs.acf.hhs.gov/school-readiness/article/news-you-can-use -early-science-learning-infants-toddlers

Moomaw, S., & Davis, J. A. (2010). STEM Comes to Preschool. *Young Children, 65*(5). https://www .researchgate.net/publication/292035679_STEM_comes_to_preschool

National Association for the Education of Young Children. (2009). *Young Children, 64*(6). [November 2009 issue focused on science.] https://www.naeyc.org/resources/topics/science

National Institute of Environmental Health Sciences. (n.d.). *Science—How it works.* https://kids.niehs .nih.gov/topics/how-science-works/index.htm

Patrick, H., Mantzicopoulos, P. Y., & Samarapungavan, A. (2009). Reading, writing, and conduct-ing inquiry about science in kindergarten. *Young Children, 64*(6). https://www.researchgate.net /publication/257981023_Reading_writing_and_conducting_inquiry_about_science_in_kindergarten

Books

Ashbrook, P. (2003). *Science is simple: Over 250 activities for preschoolers.* Gryphon House.

Counsell, S., Escalada, L., Geiken, R., Sander, M., Uhlenberg, J., Meeteren, B. V., Yoshizawa, S., & Zan, B. (2016). *STEM learning with young children: Inquiry teaching with ramps and pathways.* National Association for the Education of Young Children.

Dziengel, A. (2018). *STEAM play & learn: 20 Fun step-by-step preschool projects about science, technology, engineering, arts, and math!* Walter Foster Jr.

Editors of Teaching Young Children. (2015). *Exploring math and science in preschool.* The preschool teacher's library of playful practice set. National Association for the Education of Young Children.

Gelman, R., Brenneman, K., MacDonald, G., & Roman, M. (2009). *Preschool pathways to science.* Brookes Publishing Co.

Heroman, C. (2017). *Making and tinkering with STEM: Solving design challenges with young children.* National Association for the Education of Young Children.

Shillady, A. (2013). *Spotlight on young children: Exploring science.* National Association for the Education of Young Children.

Activities and Ideas to Try

Arkansas Child Development and Early Learning Standards. (2018). Science and technology. In *Strategies and activities: Infant toddler.* https://ecep.uark.edu/_resources/pdf_other/06_division_materials/strategies_activities_infant_toddler2018.pdf

Education.com. (n.d.). *Preschool science activities and experiments.* https://www.education.com/activity/preschool/science

Education.com. (n.d.). *Preschool science lesson plans.* https://www.education.com/lesson-plans/preschool/science

Fun Learning for Kids. (n.d.). *30 Science activities for preschoolers that are totally awesome.* https://funlearningforkids.com/science-activities-preschoolers

Hands On As We Grow. (n.d.). *Science activities for kids.* https://handsonaswegrow.com/kids-activities/learning-activities/science

Holly. (2020, September 27). 15 Fun science activities for kids. *Kids Activities Blog.* https://kidsactivitiesblog.com/50127/fun-science-activities

JumpStart. (n.d.). *Online science resources.* https://www.jumpstart.com/parents/resources/science-resources

Learning 4 Kids. (n.d.). *Science.* https://www.learning4kids.net/category/science

Levin, V. (n.d.). Science center. *Pre-K Pages.* https://www.pre-kpages.com/tag/science-center

National Association for the Education of Young Children. (2016, June 14). Supporting the scientific thinking and inquiry of toddlers and preschoolers through play. *Smithsonian National Air and Space Museum.* https://scienceinprek.si.edu/resource/document/naeyc-supporting-scientific-thinking-and-inquiry-toddlers-and-preschoolers-through

Play to Learn Preschool. (n.d.). *Learning center: Science.* https://playtolearnpreschool.us/category/science

Play to Learn Preschool. (n.d.). Science experiments—Preschool. *Pinterest.* https://www.pinterest.com/PlayToLearnPS/science-experiments-preschool

Preschool Learning Online. *Science activities for preschoolers.* https://www.preschoollearningonline.com/science-activities-for-preschoolers.html

Teaching 2 and 3 Year Olds. (n.d.). *Toddler science.* https://teaching2and3yearolds.com/category/science/toddler-science

Videos

PBS Learning Media. (n.d.). *Science* [Video series]. https://www.pbslearningmedia.org/science

ZERO TO THREE. (n.d.). *Everyday fun with science: Let's talk about STEM Video* [Video]. https://www.zerotothree.org/resources/1573-everyday-fun-with-science-let-s-talk-about-stem-video

Sensory

Articles and Readings

Howe, M. B., Brittain, L. A., & McCathren, R. B. (2004). Meeting the sensory needs of young children in classrooms. *Young Exceptional Children, 8*(1). https://www.researchgate.net/publication/234559569 _Meeting_the_Sensory_Needs_of_Young_Children_in_Classrooms

Lynch, S. A., & Simpson, C. G. (2004). Sensory processing: Meeting individual needs using the seven senses. *Young Exceptional Children, 7*(4). https://www.researchgate.net/publication/249836322 _Sensory_Processing_Meeting_Individual_Needs_Using_the_Seven_Senses

Not Just Cute with Amanda Morgan. (2009, February 11). *How to find sensory materials on the cheap.* https://notjustcute.com/2009/02/11/how-to-find-sensory-materials-on-the-cheap

Thompson, S. D., & Rain, K. W. (2008). Learning about sensory integration dysfunction: Strategies to meet young children's sensory needs at home. *Young Exceptional Children, 12*(2). https://www.researchgate .net/publication/249836110_Learning_About_Sensory_Integration_Dysfunction_Strategies_to _Meet_Young_Children%27s_Sensory_Needs_at_Home

Thompson, S. D., & Raisor, J. M. (2013). Meeting the sensory needs of young children. *Young Children, 68*(2). https://www.researchgate.net/publication/289814027_Meeting_the_sensory_needs_of _young_children

Activities and Ideas to Try

Cherry, M. (n.d.). *40 Plus awesome sensory play activities for babies and toddlers.* https://mericherry .com/2015/02/03/sensory-play-babies-toddlers

Growing a Jeweled Rose. (n.d.). *Sensory play activities for babies.* https://www.growingajeweledrose .com/2013/04/sensory-activities-potato-flakes.html

Hands On As We Grow. (n.d.). *25 Sensory activities for kids.* https://handsonaswegrow.com/sensory -activities-for-kids

Learning 4 Kids. (n.d.). *List of sensory play activities.* https://www.learning4kids.net/play-categories /list-of-sensory-play-ideas

Levin, V. (n.d.). Sensory bins. *Pre-K Pages.* https://www.pre-kpages.com/category/sensory-bins

Play to Learn Preschool. (n.d.). *Non-food sensory bin ideas for preschoolers.* https://playtolearnpreschool .us/category/sensory

Teaching 2 and 3 Year Olds. (n.d.). *Sensory bins.* https://teaching2and3yearolds.com/category/sensory -bins

Technology (Growing and Ready levels only)

Articles and Readings

Judge, S. (2001). Integrating computer technology within early childhood classrooms. *Young Exceptional Children, 5*(1). https://www.researchgate.net/publication/234642140_Integrating_Computer _Technology_Within_Early_Childhood_Classrooms

Moomaw, S., & Davis, J. A. (2010). STEM comes to preschool. *Young Children, 65*(5). https://www .researchgate.net/publication/292035679_STEM_comes_to_preschool

National Association for the Education of Young Children and Fred Rogers Center for Early Learning and Children's Media at Saint Vincent College. (2012). *Joint position statement: Technology and interactive media as tools in early childhood programs serving children from birth through age 8.* https://www.naeyc .org/sites/default/files/globally-shared/downloads/PDFs/resources/topics/PS_technology_WEB.pdf

Pecaski McLennan, D. (2017). Creating coding stories and games. *Teaching Young Children, 10*(3). https://www.naeyc.org/resources/pubs/tyc/feb2017/creating-coding-stories-and-games

Books

Counsell, S., Escalada, L., Geiken, R., Sander, M., Uhlenberg, J., Meeteren, B. V., Yoshizawa, S., & Zan, B. (2015). *STEM learning with young children: Inquiry teaching with ramps and pathways.* National Association for the Education of Young Children.

Donohue, C. (2014). *Technology and digital media in the early years: Tools for teaching and learning.* Routledge.

Donohue, C. (2016). *Family engagement in the digital age: Early childhood educators as media mentors.* National Association for the Education of Young Children.

Heroman, C. (2017). *Making and tinkering with STEM: Solving design challenges with young children.* National Association for the Education of Young Children.

Parette, H. P., & Blum, C. (2013). *Instructional technology in early childhood.* Brookes Publishing Co.

Sadao, K. C., & Robinson, N. B. (2010). *Assistive technology for young children: Creating inclusive learning environments.* Brookes Publishing Co.

Shillady, A., & Muccio, L. S. (2012). *Spotlight on young children and technology.* National Association for the Education of Young Children.

Stone-MacDonald, A., Wendell, K. B., Douglass, A., & Love, M. L. (2015). *Engaging young engineers: Teaching problem-solving skills through STEM.* Brookes Publishing Co.

Activities and Ideas to Try

ABCmouse.com. (n.d.). *Full online curriculum for children ages 2–8.* https://www.abcmouse.com/abt/homepage?8a08850bc2=T410032292.1595259042.8049

Arkansas Child Development and Early Learning Standards. (2018). Science and technology. In *Strategies and activities: Infant toddler.* https://ecep.uark.edu/_resources/pdf_other/06_division_materials/strategies_activities_infant_toddler2018.pdf

Colorín Colorado. (n.d.). *For families: Technology at home.* https://www.colorincolorado.org/technology-home

Early Childhood Teacher. (n.d.). *ECE technology: 10 Trending tools for teachers.* https://www.earlychildhoodteacher.org/blog/ece-technology-10-trending-tools-for-teachers

National Association for the Education of Young Children. (n.d.). *Technology and young children: Online resources and position statement.* https://www.naeyc.org/resources/topics/technology-and-media/resources

Videos

Colorado Department of Education. (n.d.). Results matter video library: iPads in early childhood [Video series]. https://www.cde.state.co.us/resultsmatter/RMVideoSeries_iPadsInEarlyChildhood

Writing

Articles and Readings

Baghban, M. (2007). Scribbles, labels, and stories: The role of drawing in the development of writing. *Young Children, 62*(1). https://www.researchgate.net/publication/234723247_Scribbles_Labels_and_Stories_The_Role_of_Drawing_in_the_Development_of_Writing

Early Childhood Teacher. (n.d.). *How to teach children to be successful writers.* https://www.earlychildhoodteacher.org/blog/how-to-teach-children-to-be-successful-writers

Love, A., Burns, M. S., & Buell, M. J. (2007). Writing: Empowering literacy. *Young Children, 62*(1). https://www.researchgate.net/publication/234757182_Writing_Empowering_Literacy

Not Just Cute with Amanda Morgan. (2010, August 27). *The write way to read.* https://notjustcute.com/2010/08/27/the-write-way-to-read

Books

Neuman, S. B., Copple, C., & Bredekamp, S. (2000). *Learning to read and write: Developmentally appropriate practices for young children.* National Association for the Education of Young Children.

Schickedanz, J. A., & Casbergue, R. (2009). *Writing in preschool: Learning to orchestrate meaning and marks.* National Association for the Education of Young Children.

Schickedanz, J. A., & Collins, M. F. (2012). *So much more than ABCs: The early phases of reading and writing.* National Association for the Education of Young Children.

Activities and Ideas to Try

Cincinnati Children's Blog. (2013, April 13). *5 Pre-writing activities for your 3-year-old.* https://blog.cincinnatichildrens.org/learning-and-growing/pre-writing-activities

Education.com. *Preschool writing.* https://www.education.com/resources/preschool/writing

Hanke, H. (2019, January 26). Fun activities to promote writing skills. *BabyCenter.* https://www.babycenter.com/0_fun-activities-to-promote-writing-skills_64524.bc

Levin, V. (n.d.). Writing center for preschool and pre-K. *Pre-K Pages.* https://www.pre-kpages.com/writing_center

National Writing Project. (n.d.). *Resources.* https://archive.nwp.org/cs/public/print/doc/resources.csp

Reading Rockets. (n.d.). *Writing.* https://www.readingrockets.org/teaching/reading-basics/writing

Thayer, A. (n.d.). 10 Pre-writing activities for preschoolers. *Teaching Mama.* https://teachingmama.org/prewriting-activities-for-preschoolers

The OT Toolbox. (n.d.). *Handwriting.* https://www.theottoolbox.com/handwriting

U.S. Department of Education. (n.d.). 25 Activities for reading and writing fun. *Reading Rockets.* https://www.readingrockets.org/article/25-activities-reading-and-writing-fun

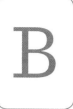

B

AEPS®-3 Skills Matrix

APPENDIX B: AEPS-3 SKILLS MATRIX

Fine Motor

AEPS-3 Test Item

AEPS-3 Test Item	Writing	Technology	Sensory	Science	Nap & Sleep	Music & Movement	Meals & Snacks	Math	Field Trips	Dressing	Dramatic Play	Diapering, Toileting, & Handwashing	Circle Time	Block Play	Bath Time	Art	Arrival & Departure	Active & Outdoor Play
A. Reach, Grasp, and Release																		
1. Makes directed batting or swiping movements with each hand					B	B			B	B		B	B	B	B	B	B	B
1.1 Brings hands together near midline						B	B		B	B		B	B	B	B	B	B	B
1.2 Makes directed movements with arms			B		B	B			B	B		B	B	B	B	B		B
FS 1.2a Child makes nondirected movements with arms.							B		B		B	B	B	B	B	B		B
2. Grasps pea-size object						B	B	B	B	B		B	B	B	B	B	B	B
FS 2a Child grasps pea-size object with either hand, using tip of index finger and thumb with hand and/or arm resting on surface for support. Thumb is to side of index finger (inferior pincer grasp).							B	B	B	B		B	B	B		B		B
2.1 Grasps hand-size object	B		B			B		B	B		B	B	B	B		B		B
FS 2.1a Child grasps hand-size object with either hand, holding object at base of index finger and thumb.							B		B									
2.2 Grasps small cylindrical object	B		B			B	B	B	B		B			B		B		
2.3 Grasps pea-size object using fingers in raking or scratching movement							B	B	B		B							
2.4 Grasps hand-size object using whole hand			B				B	B	B		B			B				
FS 2.4a Child grasps hand-size object with either hand, holding object on side of hand near little finger and against palm. Thumb is not holding object (ulnar palmar grasp).	B								B	B				B	B	B		
FS 2.4b Child briefly holds object placed in either hand.							B		B									
3. Stacks objects								B	B	B	B		B	B		B		B
FS 3a Child places small object on top of another small object with or without releasing it.									B									
3.1 Releases object into targeted space			B			B		B	B	B	B		B		B	B		B
FS 3.1a Child uses either hand to release handheld object onto or into large target while resting hand.																		

APPENDIX B: AEPS-3 SKILLS MATRIX

Fine Motor (continued)

AEPS-3 Curriculum Routine/Activity

AEPS-3 Test Item	Active & Outdoor Play	Arrival & Departure	Art	Bath Time	Block Play	Circle Time	Diapering, Toileting, & Handwashing	Dramatic Play	Dressing	Field Trips	Math	Meals & Snacks	Music & Movement	Nap & Sleep	Science	Sensory	Technology	Writing
3.2 Releases object into nondefined space	B		B	B	B			B	B	B			B			B		
FS 3.2a Child releases handheld object with either hand by pushing or pulling object against surface.																		
B. Functional Skill Use																		
1. Activates object with finger	B	B					B	B	B	B	B	B	B			B		
FS 1a Child touches or attempts to manipulate button, key, or switch to activate mechanical toy.	G	G					G	G		G	G	G	G		G	G	G	
FS 1b Child touches switch or other part of mechanical toy that produces movement or sound (e.g., child touches tail of toy animal that wags when wound up).															G		G	
1.1 Uses finger to point or touch	B		B		B	B		B	B	B			B	B		B		B
FS 1.1a Child isolates own index finger by pointing or touching (not necessarily with intent).																		
FS 1.1b Child uses thumb or fingers to poke.																		
1.2 Uses hand to activate object	B							B		B				B				
1.3 Uses fingers to explore object	B	B	G		B		G			B	B	B	B		G	G		
2. Rotates wrist to manipulate object	G		G	G	G		G	G		G	G	G	G	G	G	G		
2.1 Turns object using either hand	B	B	B	B	B			B	G	B	B	B	B	B	G	B		B
FS 2.1a Child turns hand and arm from palm-down position to face midline while holding object (e.g., child holds block in each hand with hands palm-down and turns them toward each other).	B						G	G		G	B	B	B		B	B		
FS 2.1b Child turns wrist and arm over when not holding an object (clasps fingers together and turns wrists and hand; turns one arm and hand while examining fingers).																		
3. Manipulates object with two hands, each performing different action [RS 1]	G	G	G	G	G		G	G	G	G	G	G	G	G	G	G		G
3.1 Assembles toy					G					G	G		G	G	G	G		
FS 3.1a Child takes apart toy or object that has pieces.																		

Assessment, Evaluation, and Programming System for Infants and Children, Third Edition (AEPS®-3), by Bricker, Dionne, Grisham, Johnson, Macy, Slentz, & Waddell. © 2022 Brookes Publishing Co. All rights reserved.

(page 2 of 42)

APPENDIX B: AEPS-3 SKILLS MATRIX

Fine Motor (continued)

AEPS-3 Test Item

AEPS-3 Curriculum Routine/Activity

AEPS-3 Test Item	Active & Outdoor Play	Arrival & Departure	Art	Bath Time	Block Play	Circle Time	Diapering, Toileting, & Handwashing	Dramatic Play	Dressing	Field Trips	Math	Meals & Snacks	Music & Movement	Nap & Sleep	Science	Sensory	Technology	Writing
3.2 Aligns objects	G			G	G					G	G	G		G	G			
3.3 Fits variety of shapes into corresponding spaces FS 3.3a Child places round object into corresponding space (e.g., child puts plug in drain, cup in holder, toy people in vehicles). FS 3.3b Child puts object into defined space so that object fits partially in intended space. FS 3.3c Child removes variety of shapes from corresponding spaces (e.g., child removes pieces from puzzle or form board, takes plug out of tub). FS 3.3d Child takes object out of defined space (e.g., child removes block from dump truck, cars from toy garage, cup and toothbrush from holder).				G	G					G	G			G	G			
3.4 Holds object with one hand and manipulates object or produces action with other hand FS 3.4a Child manipulates or produces action with object while adult steadies object.	B	B	B		B			B		B		B	B			B		
3.5 Transfers object from hand to hand	B	B	B		B		B	B	B	B	B		B	B		B		B
C. Mechanics of Writing																		
1. Holds writing tool using three-finger grasp to write or draw `RS 2` FS 1a Child uses three-finger grasp to hold writing tool.	R	R	R	R		R		R		R	R				R		R	R
1.1 Writes or draws using mixed strokes FS 1.1a Child draws simple shapes (e.g., circle, X).			G	G				G			G				G		G	G
1.2 Writes or draws using curved lines FS 1.2a Child makes circular or curved shape with writing tool.			G	G				G		G	G				G		G	G
1.3 Writes or draws using straight lines FS 1.3a Child makes horizontal stroke with crayon, marker, or pencil. FS 1.3b Child makes vertical stroke with crayon, marker, or pencil.			G	G				G		G	G				G		G	G
1.4 Scribbles FS 1.4a Child makes mark on paper.		G	G	G				G			G				G		G	G

APPENDIX B: AEPS-3 SKILLS MATRIX

Fine Motor (continued)

AEPS-3 Test Item

D. Use of Electronic Devices

AEPS-3 Test Item	Active & Outdoor Play	Arrival & Departure	Art	Bath Time	Block Play	Circle Time	Diapering, Toileting, & Handwashing	Dramatic Play	Dressing	Field Trips	Math	Meals & Snacks	Music & Movement	Nap & Sleep	Science	Sensory	Technology	Writing
1. Uses finger to interact with electronic device						G					G						G	G
1.1 Uses finger to interact with simple electronic game											G						G	
1.2 Uses finger to interact with touch screen																		
FS 1.2a Child uses hand or part of hand to interact with touch screen.		B																

Assessment, Evaluation, and Programming System for Infants and Children, Third Edition (AEPS®-3), by Bricker, Dionne, Grisham, Johnson, Macy, Slentz, & Waddell. © 2022 Brookes Publishing Co. All rights reserved.

(page 4 of 42)

APPENDIX B: AEPS-3 SKILLS MATRIX

Gross Motor

AEPS-3 Test Item

A. Body Control and Weight Transfer

AEPS-3 Test Item	Active & Outdoor Play	Arrival & Departure	Art	Bath Time	Block Play	Circle Time	Diapering, Toileting, & Handwashing	Dramatic Play	Dressing	Field Trips	Math	Meals & Snacks	Music & Movement	Nap & Sleep	Science	Sensory	Technology	Writing
1. Turns head, moves arms, and kicks legs independently of each other	B	B			B		B		B	B			B			B		
1.1 Kicks legs	B			B	B		B		B	B			B					
FS 1.1a Child kicks both legs together.																		
1.2 Waves arms	B			B	B				B	B			B					
1.3 Turns head side to side	B	B		B	B					B			B	B		B		
2. Puts weight on one hand or arm while reaching with opposite hand	B	B										B				B		
2.1 Remains propped on extended arms with head lifted	B											B				B		
FS 2.1a Child assumes swimming posture with weight primarily on abdomen with arms and legs stretched out above weight-bearing surface.																		
2.2 Remains propped on nonextended forearms with head lifted	B				B					B		B				B		
FS 2.2a Child lifts head and shoulders off surface when lying on stomach.																		
FS 2.2b Child uses arms to propel body backward when lying on stomach.																		
FS 2.2c Child lifts head off surface when lying on stomach.																		
3. Rolls from back to stomach		B			B				B	B				B				
3.1 Rolls from stomach to back					B					B				B				
3.2 Rolls from back or stomach to side		B			B				B	B				B				
FS 3.2a Child rolls from side to back.																		
FS 3.2b When lying on stomach or back, child positions self on verge of rolling in direction of one extended arm with face turned toward extended arm.																		

APPENDIX B: AEPS-3 SKILLS MATRIX

Gross Motor (continued)

AEPS-3 Curriculum Routine/Activity

AEPS-3 Test Item	Writing	Technology	Sensory	Science	Nap & Sleep	Music & Movement	Meals & Snacks	Math	Field Trips	Dressing	Dramatic Play	Diapering, Toileting, & Handwashing	Circle Time	Block Play	Bath Time	Art	Arrival & Departure	Active & Outdoor Play
4. Assumes balanced sitting position	B		B			B	B		B	B			B	B	B		B	B
FS 4a When standing, child lowers body, bends knees, and shifts weight backward to sitting position.																		
FS 4b When on hands and knees, child rotates body while extending and pushing with arms and shifts weight to sitting position.																		
FS 4c When on hands and knees, child shifts weight to lean back and sit on legs, then extends legs out in front to sit on buttocks.																		
FS 4d When in side-lying position, child moves to sitting position by bending at waist while extending and pushing with arms, bearing weight on hips to raise body off ground.																		
FS 4e When sitting, child leans to left and right, then regains balanced, upright sitting position.																		
4.1 Assumes hands-and-knees position from sitting			B			B			B				B	B	B		B	B
4.2 Regains balanced, upright sitting position after reaching across body			B			B	B		B				B	B	B		B	B
4.3 Regains balanced, upright sitting position after leaning left, right, and forward			B			B	B		B				B	B	B		B	B
FS 4.3a When sitting, child leans forward, then regains balanced, upright sitting position.																		
4.4 Sits balanced without support			B			B	B		B	B	B		B	B	B	B	B	B
4.5 Sits balanced using hands for support						B			B	B	B		B	B	B	B	B	B
4.6 Holds head in midline when sitting supported	B		B			B	B		B	B	B		B	B	B	B	B	B
FS 4.6a When sitting in supported position, child lifts head momentarily.																		
FS 4.6b When sitting in supported position, child holds upper back straight.																		
5. Gets out of chair	B						B	B	B	B	B					B	B	B
5.1 Sits down in chair	B						B	B	B	B	B					B	B	B
5.2 Maintains sitting position in chair	B						B	B	B	B	B					B	B	B

APPENDIX B: AEPS-3 SKILLS MATRIX

Gross Motor (continued)

AEPS-3 Test Item

B. Movement and Coordination

AEPS-3 Test Item	Active & Outdoor Play	Arrival & Departure	Art	Bath Time	Block Play	Circle Time	Diapering, Toileting, & Handwashing	Dramatic Play	Dressing	Field Trips	Math	Meals & Snacks	Music & Movement	Nap & Sleep	Science	Sensory	Technology	Writing
1. Creeps forward using alternating arm and leg movements	B	B	B							B		B						
FS 1a Child reaches with one arm while maintaining weight on other hand and both knees.																		
FS 1b Child moves under obstacles.																		
1.1 Rocks while in creeping position	B	B	B		B					B								
1.2 Assumes creeping position	B	B			B					B								
1.3 Crawls forward on stomach	B	B			B					B						B		
1.4 Pivots on stomach	B	B								B						B		
2. Stoops and regains balanced standing position	B	B	B		B	B		B	B	B		B	B			B		
FS 2a Child regains standing position after squatting or stooping by using support (e.g., furniture, wall, person).																		
2.1 Rises from sitting to standing position	B	B	B		B	B		B	B	B		B	B			B		
FS 2.1a Child leans forward from sitting position, bears weight on hands, and shifts weight from buttocks to knees.																		
2.2 Stands unsupported	B	B	B		B			B	B	B	B		B			B		
FS 2.2a Child stands bearing own full weight with one-hand support.																		
FS 2.2b Child stands bearing own full weight with two-hand support.																		
2.3 Pulls to standing position	B	B	B		B			B	B	B		B	B	B		B		
FS 2.3a Child uses support to pull up one foot from kneeling position by shifting weight to one foot and one knee.																		
2.4 Pulls to kneeling position		B			B			B						B		B		

Assessment, Evaluation, and Programming System for Infants and Children, Third Edition (AEPS®-3), by Bricker, Dionne, Grisham, Johnson, Macy, Slentz, & Waddell. © 2022 Brookes Publishing Co. All rights reserved.

APPENDIX B: AEPS-3 SKILLS MATRIX

Gross Motor (*continued*)

AEPS-3 Curriculum Routine/Activity

AEPS-3 Test Item	Active & Outdoor Play	Arrival & Departure	Art	Bath Time	Block Play	Circle Time	Diapering, Toileting, & Handwashing	Dramatic Play	Dressing	Field Trips	Math	Meals & Snacks	Music & Movement	Nap & Sleep	Science	Sensory	Technology	Writing
3. Walks avoiding people, furniture, or objects	G	G	G		G	G	G	G	G	G		G	G	G	G			G
3.1 Walks without support	B	B	B		B	B	B	B	B	B		B	B	B				B
FS 3.1a Child walks unsupported for short distance and changes direction without falling.	G	G	G		G	G	G	G	G	G		G	G	G	G		G	G
FS 3.1b Child walks unsupported for short distance without falling.	B	B	B		B	B	B	B	B	B		B	B	B				
3.2 Walks with one-hand support	B	B	B		B	B	B	B	B	B		B	B	B				B
3.3 Walks with two-hand support	B	B	B		B	B	B	B	B	B		B	B	B				B
3.4 Cruises	B	B	B		B					B		B						
FS 3.4a Child rises from sitting to standing position with support.																		
4. Alternates feet going up and down stairs	G	G								G	G				G	G		G
FS 4a Child walks up and down stairs without support. Child does not alternate feet.	G	G									G				G	G		G
4.1 Walks up and down stairs using support	G	G								G	G				G	G		G
FS 4.1a Child walks up stairs holding rail or wall with one hand.																		
FS 4.1b Child walks up stairs using two-hand support.																		
4.2 Moves up and down stairs	G	G					G			G	G				G	G		G
FS 4.2a Child moves up stairs.																		
FS 4.2b Child climbs onto adult-size furniture (e.g., chair, couch, bed) or low play structure.	G	G							G	G					G	G		G
4.3 Gets up and down from low structure	G	G	G				G		G	G		G	G		G	G		G
FS 4.3a Child moves over obstacles.																		
FS 4.3b Child climbs onto low, stable structure (e.g., low step, raised platform).																		
FS 4.3c Child climbs down from adult-size furniture (e.g., chair, couch, bed) or low play structure.																		
5. Runs while avoiding people, furniture, or other objects	G	G			G					G					G			G
FS 5a Child turns corner while running.	G	G								G								
FS 5b Child stops and starts again while running.																		

APPENDIX B: AEPS-3 SKILLS MATRIX

Gross Motor (continued)

AEPS-3 Test Item

AEPS-3 Test Item	Active & Outdoor Play	Arrival & Departure	Art	Bath Time	Block Play	Circle Time	Diapering, Toileting, & Handwashing	Dramatic Play	Dressing	Field Trips	Math	Meals & Snacks	Music & Movement	Nap & Sleep	Science	Sensory	Technology	Writing
5.1 Runs	G	G								G					G		G	
5.2 Walks fast	G	G		G						G			G		G		G	
6. Jumps forward **RS 3**	G			G			G			G			G		G		G	
FS 6a Child jumps forward, landing with one foot at a time.																		
6.1 Jumps up and down in place	G									G	G		G		G		G	
FS 6.1a Child bends at knees, rises up on feet or toes, and jumps up with one foot leading.																		
FS 6.1b Child bends at knees and rises up on toes while feet remain on ground (i.e., child "jumps up" without feet leaving ground).																		
6.2 Jumps down from low structure	G									G					G			
FS 6.2a Child step-jumps or hops (leads with one foot) from low, stable structure to supporting surface.																		
6.3 Jumps down with support	B									B								
7. Skips **RS 4**	R	R								R			R		R	R	R	
7.1 Gallops	R	R								R			R		R	R	R	
7.2 Hops forward on one foot	R	R		R						R	R		R		R	R	R	R
FS 7.2a Child balances on one foot.																		
C. Active Play																		
1. Swings bat, club, or stick to strike stationary object	R									R					R	R		
1.1 Bounces ball with one hand	R									R	R				R	R		
1.2 Bounces ball with two hands	G									G	G				G	G		
1.3 Catches ball	G									G	G				G	G		
FS 1.3a When large object is tossed to child, child stretches out two arms in front.																		

(page 9 of 42)

Assessment, Evaluation, and Programming System for Infants and Children, Third Edition (AEPS®-3), by Bricker, Dionne, Grisham, Johnson, Macy, Slentz, & Waddell. © 2022 Brookes Publishing Co. All rights reserved.

APPENDIX B: AEPS-3 SKILLS MATRIX

Gross Motor *(continued)*

AEPS-3 Curriculum Routine/Activity

AEPS-3 Test Item	Active & Outdoor Play	Arrival & Departure	Art	Bath Time	Block Play	Circle Time	Diapering, Toileting, & Handwashing	Dramatic Play	Dressing	Field Trips	Math	Meals & Snacks	Music & Movement	Nap & Sleep	Science	Sensory	Technology	Writing
1.4 Kicks ball																		
FS 1.4a When object is in front of child's feet, child walks into object and moves object forward (e.g., child walks into large foam block to move it forward).	G									G					G	G		
FS 1.4b Child kicks ball or similar object while holding onto support (e.g., adult's leg, wall, railing).																		
1.5 Throws ball overhand at target with one hand	G									G	G				G	G		
1.6 Throws or rolls ball at target with two hands	B				B					B	B					B		
FS 1.6a Child throws object forward with one or two hands, not necessarily at target.	G				G					G	G				G	G		
FS 1.6b Child flings object with one hand.																		
FS 1.6c Child rolls ball, not necessarily at target.																		
FS 1.6d Child moves ball forward (e.g., bats at it).																		
2. Uses hands to hang on play equipment with bars `RS 5`	R									R					R			
2.1 Moves swing back and forth	R									R	R							
2.2 Climbs play equipment	G									G					G			
FS 2.2a Child climbs play equipment without alternating arms and legs in coordinated fashion.																		
FS 2.2b Child moves up incline.																		
2.3 Goes down small slide	G									G	G				G			
FS 2.3a Child moves down incline.																		
3. Rides and steers bicycle	R									R					R			
3.1 Pedals and steers bicycle with training wheels	G									G					G			
3.2 Pedals and steers tricycle	G									G					G			
FS 3.2a While sitting on tricycle with feet on pedals, child pedals tricycle forward and backward.																		

(page 10 of 42)

Assessment, Evaluation, and Programming System for Infants and Children, Third Edition (AEPS®-3), by Bricker, Dionne, Grisham, Johnson, Macy, Slentz, & Waddell. © 2022 Brookes Publishing Co. All rights reserved.

APPENDIX B: AEPS-3 SKILLS MATRIX

Gross Motor (continued)

AEPS-3 Test Item

AEPS-3 Test Item	Active & Outdoor Play	Arrival & Departure	Art	Bath Time	Block Play	Circle Time	Diapering, Toileting, & Handwashing	Dramatic Play	Dressing	Field Trips	Math	Meals & Snacks	Music & Movement	Nap & Sleep	Science	Sensory	Technology	Writing
3.3 Pushes riding toy with feet while steering	B G							B G		B G								
FS 3.3a While sitting on riding toy with feet on surface, child pushes forward with feet.																		
FS 3.3b While sitting on riding toy with feet on surface, child pushes backward with feet.																		
3.4 Sits on riding toy or in wagon while in motion	B	B						B		B								

Assessment, Evaluation, and Programming System for Infants and Children, Third Edition (AEPS®-3), by Bricker, Dionne, Grisham, Johnson, Macy, Slentz, & Waddell. © 2022 Brookes Publishing Co. All rights reserved.

APPENDIX B: AEPS-3 SKILLS MATRIX

Adaptive

AEPS-3 Test Item

A. Eating and Drinking

AEPS-3 Test Item	Active & Outdoor Play	Arrival & Departure	Art	Bath Time	Block Play	Circle Time	Diapering, Toileting, & Handwashing	Dramatic Play	Dressing	Field Trips	Math	Meals & Snacks	Music & Movement	Nap & Sleep	Science	Sensory	Technology	Writing
1. Uses lips to take semisolid foods off eating utensil										B		B						
1.1 Swallows semisolid foods										B		B						
1.2 Swallows liquids										B		B		B				
2. Eats foods from variety of food groups with variety of textures										G		G			G	G		
2.1 Eats hard and chewy foods										G		G			G	G		
2.2 Eats crisp foods										B		B				B		
2.3 Eats soft and dissolvable foods										B		B				B		
3. Eats with eating utensils										G		G			G	G		
3.1 Brings food to mouth with eating utensil										R		R			R	R		
FS 3.1a Child eats by spearing food with utensil (e.g., fork, chopsticks).										G		G			G	G		
FS 3.1b Child eats by scooping food with utensil (e.g., spoon, naan, fork, tortilla).																		
3.2 Eats with fingers										B		B				B		
3.3 Accepts food presented on eating utensils										B		B						
4. Drinks from open-mouth container										G		G			G	G		
4.1 Drinks from cup with spouted lid	B									B		B		B				
4.2 Drinks from container held by adult	B									B		B		B				
FS 4.2a Child drinks from cup using some lip closure on rim of container.																		

Assessment, Evaluation, and Programming System for Infants and Children, Third Edition (AEPS®-3), by Bricker, Dionne, Grisham, Johnson, Macy, Slentz, & Waddell. © 2022 Brookes Publishing Co. All rights reserved.

APPENDIX B: AEPS-3 SKILLS MATRIX

Adaptive (continued)

AEPS-3 Test Item

AEPS-3 Curriculum Routine/Activity

AEPS-3 Test Item	Active & Outdoor Play	Arrival & Departure	Art	Bath Time	Block Play	Circle Time	Diapering, Toileting, & Handwashing	Dramatic Play	Dressing	Field Trips	Math	Meals & Snacks	Music & Movement	Nap & Sleep	Science	Sensory	Technology	Writing
5. Uses culturally appropriate social dining skills (RS 6)								R		R		R						
5.1 Puts appropriate amount of food in mouth, chews, and swallows before taking another bite										G		G				G		
5.2 Takes in appropriate amount of liquid and returns cup to surface										R		R				R		
6. Prepares food for eating										G		G				G		
6.1 Pours liquid into variety of containers				G						G		G			G	G		
6.2 Serves food with utensil										G		G				G		
B. Personal Care Routines																		
1. Carries out all toileting functions							R			R								
1.1 Indicates need to use toilet	G	G		G			G			G				G				
1.2 Has bowel and bladder control	G	G		G			G			G				G				
FS 1.2a Child sits on toilet or potty chair regularly and accomplishes bowel and bladder functions some of the time.																		
FS 1.2b Child sits on toilet or potty chair regularly without accomplishing bowel or bladder function.																		
1.3 Indicates awareness of soiled and wet pants or diapers	G	G		G			G			G				G				
2. Bathes and dries self				R						R		G		G		R		
FS 2a Child cooperates with bathing.																		
2.1 Washes and dries face				G			G									G		
2.2 Washes and dries hands		G										G		G	G	G		G

Assessment, Evaluation, and Programming System for Infants and Children, Third Edition (AEPS®-3), by Bricker, Dionne, Grisham, Johnson, Macy, Slentz, & Waddell. © 2022 Brookes Publishing Co. All rights reserved.

APPENDIX B: AEPS-3 SKILLS MATRIX

Adaptive (*continued*)

AEPS-3 Curriculum Routine/Activity

AEPS-3 Test Item	Active & Outdoor Play	Arrival & Departure	Art	Bath Time	Block Play	Circle Time	Diapering, Toileting, & Handwashing	Dramatic Play	Dressing	Field Trips	Math	Meals & Snacks	Music & Movement	Nap & Sleep	Science	Sensory	Technology	Writing
3. Completes all steps for personal hygiene, including brushing teeth, combing hair, and wiping nose				R					R	R		R		R		R		
FS 3a Child completes all steps for brushing teeth.																		
FS 3b Child completes all steps for brushing or combing hair.																		
FS 3c Child completes all steps for using tissue to clean nose.																		
3.1 Completes some steps to brush teeth, comb hair, and wipe nose				G								G		G		G		
FS 3.1a Child completes some steps for using tissue to clean nose.																		
FS 3.1a.1 Child wipes nose.																		
FS 3.1a.2 Child blows nose when adult wipes it.																		
FS 3.1a.3 Child tolerates adult wiping nose.																		
FS 3.1b Child completes some steps for brushing teeth.																		
FS 3.1b.1 Child moves toothbrush around in mouth with bristles briefly contacting teeth.																		
FS 3.1b.2 Child puts toothbrush in mouth and chews on bristles.																		
FS 3.1b.3 Child tolerates adult lightly brushing teeth and gums.																		
FS 3.1b.4 Child tolerates rubber tip of toothbrush or adult's finger covered with cloth moving over gums and teeth.																		
FS 3.1b.5 Child opens mouth on request.																		
FS 3.1c Child completes some steps for brushing or combing hair.																		
FS 3.1c.1 Child cooperates when adult brushes or combs hair.																		

C. Dressing and Undressing

AEPS-3 Test Item	Active & Outdoor Play	Arrival & Departure	Art	Bath Time	Block Play	Circle Time	Diapering, Toileting, & Handwashing	Dramatic Play	Dressing	Field Trips	Math	Meals & Snacks	Music & Movement	Nap & Sleep	Science	Sensory	Technology	Writing
1. Undresses self by removing all clothing		R		R					R					R		R		
1.1 Unfastens clothing		R		R			R	R	R							R		R
1.2 Takes off pullover clothing over head		G	G	G				G	G			G		G		G		G
FS 1.2a Child removes pullover clothing part way.		R	R	R				R	R			R		R		R		R
FS 1.2b Child indicates desire to remove pullover clothing.																		

Assessment, Evaluation, and Programming System for Infants and Children, Third Edition (AEPS®-3), by Bricker, Dionne, Grisham, Johnson, Macy, Slentz, & Waddell. © 2022 Brookes Publishing Co. All rights reserved.

APPENDIX B: AEPS-3 SKILLS MATRIX

Adaptive *(continued)*

AEPS-3 Curriculum Routine/Activity

AEPS-3 Test Item	Writing	Technology	Sensory	Science	Nap & Sleep	Music & Movement	Meals & Snacks	Math	Field Trips	Dressing	Dramatic Play	Diapering, Toileting, & Handwashing	Circle Time	Block Play	Bath Time	Art	Arrival & Departure	Active & Outdoor Play
1.3 Takes off front-opening coat, jacket, or shirt	G		G	G						G	G				G	G	G	
FS 1.3a Child removes coat, jacket, or shirt part way.																		
FS 1.3b Child indicates desire to remove coat, jacket, or shirt.																		
1.4 Takes off pants			G		G					G	G	G			G			B
FS 1.4a Child removes pants part way.																		
FS 1.4b Child indicates desire to remove pants.																		
1.5 Takes off shoes					B					B	B							B
FS 1.5a Child removes shoes part way.																		
FS 1.5b Child indicates desire to remove shoes.																		
1.6 Takes off socks					B				B	B	B							
FS 1.6a Child removes socks part way.																		
FS 1.6b Child indicates desire to remove socks.																		
1.7 Takes off hat									B	B	B							B
FS 1.7a Child removes hat part way.																		
FS 1.7b Child indicates desire to remove hat.																		
2. Selects appropriate clothing and dresses self	R		R		R					R	R				R	R	R	R
2.1 Fastens clothing															R	R	R	R
FS 2.1a Child assists in fastening clothing.																		
2.2 Puts on front-opening clothing	G		G							G	G				G	G	G	
FS 2.2a Child assists in putting on front-opening clothing.																		
2.3 Puts on pullover clothing	G		G		G					G	G				G	G	G	
FS 2.3a Child assists in putting on pullover clothing.																		
2.4 Puts on pull-up clothing			G		G					G	G	G				G	G	
FS 2.4a Child assists in putting on pull-up clothing.																		

APPENDIX B: AEPS-3 SKILLS MATRIX

Adaptive (continued)

AEPS-3 Test Item	Active & Outdoor Play	Arrival & Departure	Art	Bath Time	Block Play	Circle Time	Diapering, Toileting, & Handwashing	Dramatic Play	Dressing	Field Trips	Math	Meals & Snacks	Music & Movement	Nap & Sleep	Science	Sensory	Technology	Writing
2.5 Puts on socks		G		G				G	G					G		G		
FS 2.5a Child tries to put on socks.																		
2.6 Puts on shoes		G						G	G						G	G		
FS 2.6a Child tries to put on shoes.																		
D. Personal Safety																		
1. Takes independent action to alleviate distress, discomfort, and pain	G	G		G	G	G		G	G	G	G	G	G			G		
1.1 Communicates internal distress, discomfort, or pain to adult	G	G		G	G	G	G	G	G	G	G	G	G			G		
2. Complies with common home and community safety rules	R	R	R	R	R	R	R			R	R	R	R	R	R	R	R	R
2.1 Complies with graphic or written warning signs and symbols	R	R		R	R					R		R		R	R	R	R	R
3. Takes independent action when faced with dangerous conditions or substances	R	R					R			R		R			R	R		
3.1 Responds appropriately to warnings of dangerous conditions or substances	R	G					R			G	G	G	G	R	R	R		
4. Recognizes and reports information regarding safety RS 7													R		R			
4.1 States or produces personal information to promote/maintain personal safety	R	R				R	R	R		R					R	R		R
4.2 Reports inappropriate events, actions, or language by others	R	R	R		R	R	R	R		R	R	R	R	R	R	R	R	R

AEPS-3 Curriculum Routine/Activity

(page 16 of 42)

APPENDIX B: AEPS-3 SKILLS MATRIX

Social-Emotional

AEPS-3 Test Item

A. Interactions with Adults

AEPS-3 Curriculum Routine/Activity

AEPS-3 Test Item	Active & Outdoor Play	Arrival & Departure	Art	Bath Time	Block Play	Circle Time	Diapering, Toileting, & Handwashing	Dramatic Play	Dressing	Field Trips	Math	Meals & Snacks	Music & Movement	Nap & Sleep	Science	Sensory	Technology	Writing
1. Initiates positive social behavior toward familiar adult	B	B	B	B	B	B	B		B	B		B	B	B				
1.1 Responds appropriately to familiar adult's affective tone	B	B	B	B	B	B	B		B	B		B	B	B				
1.2 Responds to familiar adult's positive social behavior	B	B	B	B	B	B	B		B	B		B	B					
FS 1.2a Child responds to familiar adult's social behavior by maintaining or continuing interaction (e.g., child knocks down block tower that adult built and waits for or helps adult to rebuild tower).																		
FS 1.2b Child shows interest in communication from familiar adult (e.g., child stops crying when adult talks soothingly, increases motor action when adult speaks playfully, looks at adult who is talking, watches adult as adult sings).																		
2. Maintains social interaction with familiar adult	B	B	B	B	B		B			B	B	B	B	B				
FS 2a Child responds to communication from familiar adult and maintains interaction (e.g., adult asks child to tell about pictures in book, and child makes vocalizations about pictures; then adult supplies words for pictures, and child vocalizes again or points to picture).																		
2.1 Initiates simple social interaction with familiar adult	B	B	B	B	B		B		B	B	B	B	B					
FS 2.1a Child assumes active role in drawing attention of or getting close to familiar adult to continue social game (e.g., child crawls after father, tugs at grandma's clothes, or climbs into mother's lap).																		
2.2 Repeats part of interactive game or action in order to continue game or action	B		B	B	B	B		B		B	B		B					
2.3 Responds to familiar game or action	B		B	B	B	B		B	B	B	B							
FS 2.3a Child interacts with familiar adult in vocally similar manner by matching patterns of vocal exchanges (e.g., child gurgles when adult stops vocalizing, child varies length of vocalizations as function of length of adult's verbalizations, child changes rhythm of vocalizations when adult sings to child).																		

APPENDIX B: AEPS-3 SKILLS MATRIX

Social-Emotional *(continued)*

AEPS-3 Curriculum Routine/Activity

AEPS-3 Test Item	Active & Outdoor Play	Arrival & Departure	Art	Bath Time	Block Play	Circle Time	Diapering, Toileting, & Handwashing	Dramatic Play	Dressing	Field Trips	Math	Meals & Snacks	Music & Movement	Nap & Sleep	Science	Sensory	Technology	Writing
3. Participates in familiar social routines with caregivers			G	G								G	G	G			G	
3.1 Initiates next step of familiar social routine		G	G	G		G	G		G			G	G	G	G			G
3.2 Follows familiar social routines with familiar adults		G	G	G	G	G	G		G	G		G	G	G	G			G
FS 3.2a Child responds to established social routines.																		
B. Social-Emotional Expression and Regulation																		
1. Responds appropriately to others' emotions	G	G		G	G	G	G	G		G		G						G
FS 1a Child responds appropriately to familiar adult's affect.																		
FS 1b Child displays affection toward familiar adult.																		
FS 1c Child returns affection modeled by adult.																		
FS 1d Child smiles in response to familiar adult.																		
FS 1e Child reacts differently to familiar and unfamiliar adults.																		
FS 1f Child stops crying in response to familiar adult (e.g., approach, vocalization, smile, appearance).																		
1.1 Identifies/labels emotions in others	G	G		G	G	G		G		G					G	G	G	G
1.2 Identifies/labels own emotions	G	G		G	G		G	G	G	G					G	G	G	G
2. Uses appropriate strategies to manage emotional states	G	G		G		G	G	G	G	G		G	G	G	G	G	G	G
FS 2a Child shows awareness of external physical needs such as being cold, hot, dirty, wet, or hurt. Child demonstrates discomfort by frowning or whining while wearing dirty or wet clothes.																		
FS 2b Child uses pacifier, own thumb, or adult's finger for nonnutritive sucking.																		
FS 2c Child can be soothed by familiar adult caregiver.																		
2.1 Responds appropriately to soothing by peer	G	G			G			G					G		G	G		G

Assessment, Evaluation, and Programming System for Infants and Children, Third Edition (AEPS®-3), by Bricker, Dionne, Grisham, Johnson, Macy, Slentz, & Waddell. © 2022 Brookes Publishing Co. All rights reserved.

APPENDIX B: AEPS-3 SKILLS MATRIX

Social-Emotional (*continued*)

AEPS-3 Curriculum Routine/Activity

AEPS-3 Test Item	Writing	Technology	Sensory	Science	Nap & Sleep	Music & Movement	Meals & Snacks	Math	Field Trips	Dressing	Dramatic Play	Diapering, Toileting, & Handwashing	Circle Time	Block Play	Bath Time	Art	Arrival & Departure	Active & Outdoor Play
2.2 Seeks comfort, closeness, or physical contact from familiar adult			B		B	B	B		B	B		B	B	B			B	B
FS 2.2a Child responds in attempt to prolong positive interaction (e.g., when mother looks away from child, child touches mother's face to get her to look back again).																		
FS 2.2b Child uses familiar adults for comfort, closeness, or physical contact.																		
FS 2.2c Child differentiates between familiar and unfamiliar adults for comfort, closeness, or physical contact.																		
2.3 Responds appropriately to soothing by adult			B		B	B	B		B	B		B	B	B			B	B
FS 2.3a Child shows interest in familiar adult's social behavior (e.g., child looks at adult when adult plays Peekaboo or smiles when adult peeks around corner).																		
3. Makes positive statements about self or accomplishments	G	G	G	G	G	G	G	G	G	G	G	G	G	G		G	G	G
3.1 Explains or shows others how to do tasks mastered	R	R	R	R	R	R	R	R	R	R	R	R	R	R	R	R	R	R
3.2 Shares accomplishment with familiar caregiver	G	G	G	G	G	G	G	G	G	G	G	G	G	G	G	G	G	G
C. Interactions with Peers																		
1. Maintains interaction with peer	G	G	G	G	G	G	G	G	G	G	G	G		G		G	G	G
1.1 Initiates social behavior toward peer	G	G	G	G	G	G	G	G	G	G	G	G		G		G	G	G
1.2 Responds appropriately to peer social behavior	G	G	G	G	G	G	G	G	G	G	G	G		G		G	G	G
FS 1.2a Child shows interest in peer's social behavior (e.g., child looks at toy offered by peer, child waves arms and smiles while watching peer on swing).																		

APPENDIX B: AEPS-3 SKILLS MATRIX

Social-Emotional (continued)

AEPS-3 Test Item	Active & Outdoor Play	Arrival & Departure	Art	Bath Time	Block Play	Circle Time	Diapering, Toileting, & Handwashing	Dramatic Play	Dressing	Field Trips	Math	Meals & Snacks	Music & Movement	Nap & Sleep	Science	Sensory	Technology	Writing
1.3 Plays near one or two peers	B	B			B			B		B	B		B			B		B
FS 1.3a Child plays near one or two peers in presence of familiar adult (e.g., child plays with Legos in proximity of teacher reading a story to a peer).																		
FS 1.3b Child observes peers or siblings (e.g., child watches older sibling playing with friend).																		
FS 1.3c Child entertains self by playing appropriately with toys.																		
2. Plans and acts out recognizable event, theme, or storyline in imaginary play	R			R	R			R	R									
FS 2a Child uses action associated with common object, but object is absent; focus of child's play is on action rather than imaginary object (e.g., child kicks imaginary ball, eats imaginary cookie, throws imaginary ball).																		
2.1 Enacts roles or identities in imaginary play	R			R	R			R	R									
FS 2.1a Child enacts typical action of familiar character or animal by using real object associated with character or animal (e.g., child sits in baby brother's chair and pretends to cry, child takes mother's keys and pretends to go bye-bye).																		
FS 2.1b Child enacts imaginary events related to daily routine activities (e.g., child pretends to sleep on bed, drink from empty cup).																		
2.2 Uses imaginary props in play	R			R	R			R		R								
FS 2.2a Child uses imaginary objects in play. `RS 8`																		
3. Maintains cooperative activity	R		R	R	R			R	R	R							R	
3.1 Initiates cooperative activity	G		G		G			G	G	G							G	
3.2 Joins others in cooperative activity	G		G		G			G	G	G							G	
3.3 Shares or exchanges objects					G			G		G	G		G		G			G
4. Maintains engagement in games with rules	R							R		R	R	R	R				R	
4.1 Knows and follows game rules	R							R		R	R	R	R				R	
4.2 Participates in game	R			R				R		R	R	R	R				R	

AEPS-3 Curriculum Routine/Activity

APPENDIX B: AEPS-3 SKILLS MATRIX

Social-Emotional (continued)

AEPS-3 Test Item

D. Independent and Group Participation

AEPS-3 Test Item		Active & Outdoor Play	Arrival & Departure	Art	Bath Time	Block Play	Circle Time	Diapering, Toileting, & Handwashing	Dramatic Play	Dressing	Field Trips	Math	Meals & Snacks	Music & Movement	Nap & Sleep	Science	Sensory	Technology	Writing
1. Interacts appropriately with others during small-group activities	RS 9	G	G	G		G	G		G		G	G	G	G		G	G		G
1.1 Interacts appropriately with materials during small-group activities			G	G	G	G	G		G		G	G	G	G		G	G	G	G
1.2 Responds appropriately to directions during small-group activities		G	G	G	G	G			G		G	G	G	G		G	G	G	G
1.3 Remains with group during small-group activities		G	G	G		G	G		G		G	G	G	G		G	G	G	G
2. Interacts appropriately with others during large-group activities	RS 10						G				G	G		G		G	G	G	G
2.1 Interacts appropriately with materials during large-group activities		G	G	G		G	G	G	G	G	G	G	G	G		G		G	G
2.2 Responds appropriately to directions during large-group activities		G	G	G		G	G	G	G	G	G	G	G	G		G		G	G
2.3 Remains with group during large-group activities		G	G			B					G	G		G		G			G
3. Initiates and completes independent activities	RS 11		G	G	G	G		G	G	G	G	G	G		G	G		G	G
3.1 Responds to request to finish activity		G		G	G	G		G		G	G	G			G	G		G	G
3.2 Responds to request to begin activity				G	G	G	G	G		G	G	G	G		G	G		G	G
3.3 Entertains self by playing with toys		B	B	B	B	B			B		B	B							B
4. Resolves conflicts using negotiation	RS 12	G	G	G		G	G	G	G	G	G	G	G	G	G			G	G
4.1 Uses strategies to resolve conflicts		G		G		G		G	G			B	G	B	G	G		G	G
4.2 Claims and defends possessions		B	G	G		G			G		B	G	B	B		G			G

APPENDIX B: AEPS-3 SKILLS MATRIX

Social-Emotional *(continued)*

AEPS-3 Test Item

E. Meeting Social Expectations

AEPS-3 Test Item		Active & Outdoor Play	Arrival & Departure	Art	Bath Time	Block Play	Circle Time	Diapering, Toileting, & Handwashing	Dramatic Play	Dressing	Field Trips	Math	Meals & Snacks	Music & Movement	Nap & Sleep	Science	Sensory	Technology	Writing
1. Meets observable physical needs in socially appropriate ways	RS 13	R	R		R	R	R	R	G	R	R	R	R	R	R	R	G		
1.1 Meets internal physical needs of hunger and thirst		G			R	G			G		G		G				R		
2. Meets accepted social norms in community settings		R	R			R	R	R	G	R	R		R	R		R		G	
2.1 Meets behavioral expectations in familiar environments		G	G	G	G	G	G	G	G		G	G	G	G	G		G	G	
2.2 Adjusts behavior based on feedback from others or environment		G	G	G	G	G	G	G	G	G	G	G	G	G	G		G	G	R
FS 2.2a Child understands how own behavior affects others.		R	G	G	G	G	R	R	R	G	R		R	R	R	R	R	R	R
3. Follows context-specific rules	RS 14	R	R	R	R	R	R	R	R		R	R	R	R	R	R	R	R	R
3.1 Seeks adult permission when appropriate		G	G	G		G	G	G	G		G			G				G	
3.2 Follows established social rules in familiar environments		G	G	G			G	G	G	G		G		G	G		G	G	G
4. Relates identifying information about self	RS 15	R	R		R	R	R	R	R		R		R	R	R	R	R	G	R
4.1 States birthday					R				R				R	R	R	R	R		R
4.2 States age				G			G		G					G			G	G	
4.3 Provides given name or nickname of self and others		G	G	G			G		G								G		

APPENDIX B: AEPS-3 SKILLS MATRIX

Social-Communication

A. Early Social Communication

AEPS-3 Test Item	Active & Outdoor Play	Arrival & Departure	Art	Bath Time	Block Play	Circle Time	Diapering, Toileting, & Handwashing	Dramatic Play	Dressing	Field Trips	Math	Meals & Snacks	Music & Movement	Nap & Sleep	Science	Sensory	Technology	Writing
1. Turns and looks toward person speaking — FS 1a Child turns and looks toward noise-producing object.	B	B	B	B	B	B	B	B	B	B		B	B			B		
1.1 Quiets to familiar voice		B	B	B	B	B			B	B		B	B	B				
2. Produces speech sounds		B	B	B	B	B	B	B	B	B		B	B			B		B
2.1 Coos and gurgles		B	B	B	B	B	B		B	B		B	B			B		
3. Engages in vocal exchanges — FS3a Child uses behaviors similar to communication skills (e.g., while awake in crib, child uses vocalizations, gestures, and expressions similar to those used to communicate).		B	B	B	B	B	B	B	B	B		B	B			B		
3.1 Vocalizes to another person expressing positive affective state	B	B	B		B	B	B	B	B	B		B	B			B		
3.2 Vocalizes to another person expressing negative affective state	B	B	B		B	B	B	B	B	B		B	B			B		
4. Uses intentional gestures, vocalizations, and objects to communicate	B	B	B		B	B	B	B	B	B	B	B	B			B		

FS 4a Child demonstrates greeting function of communication by gesturing or vocalizing (e.g., when sibling enters room, child vocalizes or uses waving gesture; adult enters room and child vocalizes or uses "up" reaching gesture).

FS 4b Child demonstrates confirmation function of communication by gesturing or vocalizing (e.g., when adult says "There's the ball," child points to ball).

FS 4c Child demonstrates comment/reply function of communication by gesturing or vocalizing (e.g., when adult asks "What happened?" child points to spilled milk).

FS 4d Child demonstrates information function of communication by gesturing or vocalizing (e.g., when adult asks "Where's your teddy?" child points to teddy bear).

FS 4e Child demonstrates attention function of communication by gesturing or vocalizing (e.g., child points to sibling jumping in swimming pool; adult says "There's Billy").

FS 4f Child demonstrates question function of communication by gesturing or vocalizing (e.g., child points to new stuffed animal; adult says "What's that?").

FS 4g Child demonstrates comment/describe function of communication by gesturing or vocalizing (e.g., child points to truck; adult says "That's a truck").

APPENDIX B: AEPS-3 SKILLS MATRIX

Social-Communication (continued)

AEPS-3 Test Item

AEPS-3 Curriculum Routine/Activity

AEPS-3 Test Item	Writing	Technology	Sensory	Science	Nap & Sleep	Music & Movement	Meals & Snacks	Math	Field Trips	Dressing	Dramatic Play	Diapering, Toileting, & Handwashing	Circle Time	Block Play	Bath Time	Art	Arrival & Departure	Active & Outdoor Play
4.1 Makes requests of others					B	B	B	B	B	B	B		B	B	B	B	B	B
4.2 Makes choices to express preferences	B		B		B	B	B	B	B	B	B		B	B	B	B	B	
4.3 Expresses desire to continue activity			B			B	B		B		B		B	B	B	B		
FS 4.3a Child reproduces action (e.g., waves arms, vocalizes, smiles) after an adult is attentive to child's initial behavior.																		
FS 4.3b Child indicates desire for adult to continue game or action by touching part of adult's body used to produce game or action (e.g., child touches adult's hand or eyes to indicate desire to continue playing Peekaboo).																		
FS 4.3c Child indicates desire to continue familiar game or action (e.g., child waves arms, bounces, vocalizes, laughs, smiles, kicks legs).																		
4.4 Expresses negation or protests			B			B	B		B		B	B	B	B	B	B	B	B
FS 4.4a Child demonstrates protest function of communication by gesturing or vocalizing displeasure (e.g., adult puts child in crib, child cries).																		
FS 4.4b Child demonstrates rejection function of communication by gesturing or vocalizing refusal (e.g., when adult puts bottle to child's mouth, child closes mouth and turns away; when adult offers child toy, child pushes toy away; when adult gives child cracker, child turns head away).																		
B. Communicative Understanding																		
1. Follows gaze to establish joint attention	B		B			B	B	B	B	B	B	B	B	B	B	B	B	B
1.1 Follows pointing gestures with eyes	B					B	B	B	B	B	B	B	B	B	G	B	B	B
1.2 Looks toward object	B					B	B	B	B	B	B	B	B	G	B	B	B	B
2. Locates common objects, people, or events	G	G	G	G		G	G	G	B	B	G	G	B	G	G	G	B	G
FS 2a Child locates common objects, people, or events in familiar pictures.																		
FS 2b Child locates common objects, people, events, or actions with contextual cues.																		
2.1 Recognizes own and familiar names						B	B		B	B	B		B			B	B	B
2.2 Responds to single-word directive						B	B		B	B	B		B			B	B	B

Assessment, Evaluation, and Programming System for Infants and Children, Third Edition (AEPS®-3), by Bricker, Dionne, Grisham, Johnson, Macy, Slentz, & Waddell. © 2022 Brookes Publishing Co. All rights reserved.

APPENDIX B: AEPS-3 SKILLS MATRIX

Social-Communication (continued)

AEPS-3 Test Item	Active & Outdoor Play	Arrival & Departure	Art	Bath Time	Block Play	Circle Time	Diapering, Toileting, & Handwashing	Dramatic Play	Dressing	Field Trips	Math	Meals & Snacks	Music & Movement	Nap & Sleep	Science	Sensory	Technology	Writing
3. Follows multistep directions without contextual cues	G	G	G	G	G	G	G	G	G	G	G	G	G	G	G	G	G	G
3.1 Follows multistep directions with contextual cues	G	G	G	G	G	G	G	G	G	G	G	G	G	G	G	G	G	G
3.2 Follows one-step direction without contextual cues	G	G	G	G	G	G	G	G	G	G	G	G	G	G	G	G	G	G
3.3 Follows one-step direction with contextual cues	G	G	G	G	G	G	G	G	G	G	G	G	G	G	G	G	G	G
FS 3.3a Child participates in verbal and gestural social routines (e.g., child responds to requests to "Come here" or "Sit down").	R	R	R	R	R	R	R	R	R	R	R	R		R	R	R	R	R
4. Responds to comprehension questions related to *why, how,* and *when*	G	G		R	G	R	R	G	R	R	R	R	G	G	G	G	G	R
4.1 Answers *who, what,* and *where* questions	G	G		G	G	G	G	G	G	G	G	G		G	G	G	G	G
FS 4.1a Child responds with vocalization or gesture to simple questions.																		

C. Communicative Expression

AEPS-3 Test Item	Active & Outdoor Play	Arrival & Departure	Art	Bath Time	Block Play	Circle Time	Diapering, Toileting, & Handwashing	Dramatic Play	Dressing	Field Trips	Math	Meals & Snacks	Music & Movement	Nap & Sleep	Science	Sensory	Technology	Writing
1. Produces multiple-word sentences to communicate	G	G	G	G	G	G	G	G	G	G	G	G	G	G	G	G	G	G
1.1 Uses two-word utterances	G	G	G	G	G	G	G	G	G	G	G	G	G	G	G	G	G	G
1.2 Uses 50 single words, signs, or symbols	G	G	G	G	G	G	G	G	G	G	G	G	G	G	G	G	G	G
1.3 Uses consistent approximations for words or signs	B	B	G	B	B	B	B	B	B	G	G	B	B	B	G	B	G	B
1.4 Uses consistent consonant-vowel combinations	B	B	G	B	B	B	G	B	B	G	G	B	G	B	G	B		B
2. Uses plural pronouns to indicate subjects, objects, and possession in multiple-word sentences	G	G	G	G	G	G	G	G	G	G	G	G	G	G	G	G	G	G
2.1 Uses irregular plural nouns in multiple-word sentences✱	G	G	G	R	G	G	G	R	G	G	G	G	G	G	G	R	G	R
2.2 Uses regular plural nouns✱	G	G	G	G	G	G	G	R	G	R	G	G	G	G	G	R	G	G

✱ This item is modified in Spanish. See Volume 2, *AEPS-3 Assessment*, Chapter 3, for details.

APPENDIX B: AEPS-3 SKILLS MATRIX

Social-Communication (continued)

AEPS-3 Curriculum Routine/Activity

AEPS-3 Test Item	Active & Outdoor Play	Arrival & Departure	Art	Bath Time	Block Play	Circle Time	Diapering, Toileting, & Handwashing	Dramatic Play	Dressing	Field Trips	Math	Meals & Snacks	Music & Movement	Nap & Sleep	Science	Sensory	Technology	Writing
3. Uses helping verbs*	G	G	G	G	G	G	G	G	G	G				G	G		G	
3.1 Uses irregular past tense of common verbs*	R	R		R	R	G	G	R	G	R	R	R	R	R	R	R	R	R
3.2 Uses regular past tense of common verbs	G	G	G	G	G	G	G	G	G	G	G	G	G	G	G	G	G	G
3.3 Uses *to be* verbs*	G	G	G	G	G	G	G	G	G	G	G	G	G	G	G	G	G	G
4. Asks questions using inverted auxiliary*	G	R	G	G	R	G	G	R	G	R	G	R		R	R	R	R	R
4.1 Asks *wh-* questions	G	G	G	G	G	G	G	G	G	G	G	G		G	G		G	G
D. Social Use of Language																		
1. Uses language to initiate and sustain social interaction RS 16	G	G	G	G	G	G	G	G	G	G	G	G		G	G	G	G	G
1.1 Follows social conventions of language	G	G		G	G	R	G	G	G	G	G	G		G	G	G	G	G
2. Provides and seeks information while conversing using words, phrases, or sentences RS 17	G	G	G	G	G	G	G	G	G	G	G	G	G		G	G	G	G
2.1 Asks questions to obtain information	G	G	G	G	G	G		G		G	G	G			G		G	G
2.2 Describes objects, people, and events as part of social exchange	G	G	G	G	G	R	G	G	G	G	G	G		R	G	G	G	G
3. Uses conversational rules when communicating with others RS 18	R	R	R	R	R	R	R	R	R	R	R	R	R	R	R	G	R	R
3.1 Uses socially appropriate physical orientation	R	R	R	R	R	R		R	R	R	R	R	R	R	R	R	R	
3.2 Varies voice to impart meaning and recognize social or environmental conditions	R	R	R	R	R	R		R	R	R	R	R	R	R	R	R	R	R

(page 26 of 42)

* This item is modified in Spanish. See Volume 2, AEPS-3 Assessment, Chapter 3, for details.

APPENDIX B: AEPS-3 SKILLS MATRIX

Social-Communication (continued)

AEPS-3 Test Item	AEPS-3 Curriculum Routine/Activity																	
	Active & Outdoor Play	Arrival & Departure	Art	Bath Time	Block Play	Circle Time	Diapering, Toileting, & Handwashing	Dramatic Play	Dressing	Field Trips	Math	Meals & Snacks	Music & Movement	Nap & Sleep	Science	Sensory	Technology	Writing
3.3 Responds to topic initiations from others	G R		G R		G R	G R		G R	G R	G R	G R	G R						
3.4 Alternates between speaker and listener roles during conversations with others	G	G	G	G	G	G	G	G	G	G	G	G		G	G	G		G
3.5 Responds to contingent questions from others	G	G	G	G	G	G	G	G	G	G	G	G		G	G	G		G

APPENDIX B: AEPS-3 SKILLS MATRIX

Cognitive

AEPS-3 Test Item	Active & Outdoor Play	Arrival & Departure	Art	Bath Time	Block Play	Circle Time	Diapering, Toileting, & Handwashing	Dramatic Play	Dressing	Field Trips	Math	Meals & Snacks	Music & Movement	Nap & Sleep	Science	Sensory	Technology	Writing
A. Sensory Exploration																		
1. Orients to events or stimulation																		
FS 1a Child displays reflexive responses to tactile events, such as rooting response and grasp.	B	B	B	B	B	B	B	B	B	B	B	B	B			B		
FS 1b Child visually follows object moving in a circular direction.																		
FS 1c Child visually follows object moving in a vertical direction.																		
FS 1d Child visually follows object moving in a horizontal direction.																		
1.1 Reacts to events or stimulation																		
FS 1.1a Child displays reflexive pupillary and blinking responses when facing bright lights.	B		B	B	B	B	B	B	B	B	B	B	B			B		
2. Combines simple actions to examine people, animals, and objects	B	B	B	B	B	B		B		B	B	B	B			B		
2.1 Uses sensory means to explore people, animals, and objects																		
FS 2.1a Child explores and plays with parts of own body (e.g., child sucks fingers or watches hands and feet).	B	B	B	B	B	B	B	B	B	B	B	B	B			B		
FS 2.1b Child explores or plays with objects that satisfy physical needs (e.g., mother's breast, nipple on bottle, pacifier, blanket, clothing).			B	B	B	B		B	B	B	B	B	B			B		
B. Imitation and Memory																		
1. Imitates novel coordinated motor actions	G	G	G	G	G	G	G	G	G	G	G	G	G		G	G	G	G
1.1 Imitates novel simple motor action not already in repertoire	B	B	B	B	B	B	B	B	B	B	B	B	B			B		B
1.2 Imitates familiar simple motor action	B	B	B	B	B	B	B	B	B	B	B	B	B			B		B
FS 1.2a Child reproduces motor action similar to, but different from, adult's modeling (e.g., adult opens and closes fingers; child waves own hand).																		
FS 1.2b Child initiates action, adult imitates child's action, and child repeats action by imitating adult (e.g., child sticks out tongue, adult imitates, child repeats action within turn-taking interaction).																		

APPENDIX B: AEPS-3 SKILLS MATRIX

Cognitive (continued)

AEPS-3 Curriculum Routine/Activity

AEPS-3 Test Item	Active & Outdoor Play	Arrival & Departure	Art	Bath Time	Block Play	Circle Time	Diapering, Toileting, & Handwashing	Dramatic Play	Dressing	Field Trips	Math	Meals & Snacks	Music & Movement	Nap & Sleep	Science	Sensory	Technology	Writing
2. Imitates novel words	B	G	G	G	G	G	G	G	G	G	G	G	G	G	G	G	G	G
2.1 Imitates novel vocalizations	B	B	R	B	B	B	B	B	B	B	B	B	B					
2.2 Imitates familiar vocalizations	B	B	R	B	B	B	B	B	B	B	B	B	B					
3. Relates past events	R	R	G	R	R	R	R	R	R	R		R	R	R	R	R	R	R
3.1 Relates recent events without contextual cues	G	G	R	G	R	G	G	G	G	G		G	G	G	G	G	G	G
3.2 Relates recent events with contextual cues	R	R	G	R	R	G	G	G	R	G			G	R	R	R		R
3.3 Relates events immediately after they occur	G	G	G	G	G	G	G	G	G	G		G	G	G	G	G	G	G
C. Conceptual Knowledge																		
1. Maintains search for object not in its usual location	R	R		R	R	R	R	R	R	R		R	R		R	R		R

2. Imitates novel words

FS 2a Child says a sound or word, adult responds with novel word that is modification of child-initiated sound or word, child imitates novel word (e.g., child says "Baba," adult responds "Bobbie," child imitates "Bobbie").

FS 2b Child says simple, familiar consonant-vowel word, adult imitates word, child repeats word by imitating adult (e.g., child says "Go," adult says "Go," child imitates "Go").

C. Conceptual Knowledge

1. Maintains search for object not in its usual location

FS 1a Child asks adult for object when object is not found in its usual location.

FS 1b Child maintains search for object in its usual location (e.g., child searches second time in toy box for favorite toy).

FS 1c Child looks for object in its usual location.

FS 1d Child looks for object in proximity of its usual location (e.g., child goes into kitchen and requests cracker, child looks for ball in corner where toys are kept).

APPENDIX B: AEPS-3 SKILLS MATRIX

Cognitive *(continued)*

AEPS-3 Curriculum Routine/Activity

AEPS-3 Test Item	Writing	Technology	Sensory	Science	Nap & Sleep	Music & Movement	Meals & Snacks	Math	Field Trips	Dressing	Dramatic Play	Diapering, Toileting, & Handwashing	Circle Time	Block Play	Bath Time	Art	Arrival & Departure	Active & Outdoor Play
1.1 Locates object in second of two hiding places		G	G	G							G			G				G
FS 1.1a After child sees object hidden first in one place, then another, child searches for object in first hiding place.																		
FS 1.1b After child sees object hidden first in one place, then another, child searches for object in first hiding place.																		
FS 1.1c Child searches for object by continuing to follow object's path after it disappears (e.g., child looks for toy train at end of tunnel through which train has disappeared).																		
FS 1.1d Child looks for hidden object where object was last seen before it disappeared (e.g., adult takes doll from child's lap and covers it with blanket, child searches for doll in lap or in adult's hand).																		
1.2 Locates hidden object							B			B	B			B	B		B	B
2. Recognizes symbols				G		G			G		G		G	G	G			G
FS 2a Child labels familiar people, actions, objects, and events in pictures.																		
FS 2b Child indicates recognition of familiar people, actions, objects, and events by pointing to, touching, or picking up picture.																		
2.1 Uses object to represent another object		G		G		G			G	G	G	G	G	G			G	G
FS 2.1a Child uses representational actions with objects (e.g., child pretends to peel and eat plastic banana).																		
FS 2.1b Child uses picture or toy to represent real object (e.g., child makes barking noise while holding picture of dog).																		
FS 2.1c Child uses functionally similar object as substitute for another object to perform game or action (e.g., child feeds doll with bottle, then takes cup and gives doll drink).																		
FS 2.1d Child uses functionally appropriate actions with objects (e.g., child pretends to talk on toy phone).																		
FS 2.1e Child differentiates actions on objects according to response of object (e.g., bangs together hard objects; rolls, rattles, or shakes round objects; chews on soft objects).																		
FS 2.1f Child uses simple motor actions on different objects.																		
FS 2.1g Child produces simple, undifferentiated action on all objects (e.g., drops or bangs objects).																		

APPENDIX B: AEPS-3 SKILLS MATRIX

Cognitive (continued)

AEPS-3 Curriculum Routine/Activity

AEPS-3 Test Item	Writing	Technology	Sensory	Science	Nap & Sleep	Music & Movement	Meals & Snacks	Math	Field Trips	Dressing	Dramatic Play	Diapering, Toileting, & Handwashing	Circle Time	Block Play	Bath Time	Art	Arrival & Departure	Active & Outdoor Play
3. Classifies using multiple attributes																		
3.1 Classifies according to function		R		R			R		R	R			R	R	G			G
FS 3.1a Child groups two functionally related objects (e.g., diaper and pin, doll and blanket).		G		G			G	G	G	G	G		G	G				R
FS 3.1b Child functionally relates one object to succession of similar objects from another class (e.g., child gives each of three dolls drink, in turn, from toy cup).	R	R	R	R			R			R	R				R	R		
3.2 Classifies according to physical attribute		G		G			G	G	G	G	G		G	G	G	G		G
FS 3.2a Child groups together two or more similar objects (e.g., child chooses toy airplanes, child chooses two spoons from drawer).																		G
3.3 Discriminates between objects or people using common attributes		G		G		G	G	G	G		G		G	G	G		G	G
FS 3.3a Child recognizes familiar object, person, or event by responding in same way to similar object, person, or event over time (e.g., child looks into all mirrors and smiles, child poses in front of camera).		G	G	G		G	G		G		G	R	G		R	R	R	R
4. Uses early conceptual comparisons																		
4.1 Identifies common concepts	G	G	G	G	G	G	G	R	G	G	G	G	G	G	G	G	G	G
FS 4.1a Child demonstrates understanding of at least six pairs of early opposite concepts by sorting, labeling, or selecting objects with appropriate quality from at least six pairs (e.g., hot/cold, top/bottom, in/out, wet/dry, full/empty, up/down, stop/go, fast/slow, clean/dirty).	R	R	R	R	R	R		R	R			R	R		R	R	R	R
4.2 Identifies concrete concepts	G		G	G	G	G	G		G	G	G		G	G	G	G	G	G

APPENDIX B: AEPS-3 SKILLS MATRIX

Cognitive *(continued)*

AEPS-3 Test Item

D. Reasoning

AEPS-3 Curriculum Routine/Activity

AEPS-3 Test Item	Active & Outdoor Play	Arrival & Departure	Art	Bath Time	Block Play	Circle Time	Diapering, Toileting, & Handwashing	Dramatic Play	Dressing	Field Trips	Math	Meals & Snacks	Music & Movement	Nap & Sleep	Science	Sensory	Technology	Writing
1. Uses object to obtain another object																		
1.1 Uses part of object or support to obtain another object	B				B			B	B			B						B
FS 1.1a Child uses object to act upon another object (e.g., child hits drum with stick or draws line with stick in wet sand).	G		B	B	B			B	B			B			G			B
FS 1.1b Child acts on part of object or support to produce visible or auditory effect (e.g., child pulls placemat and dish rattles, child pulls string and toy moves).			B	G	G			G	G			G						G
FS 1.1c Child moves own body parts to produce effect on object (e.g., child kicks crib mobile).			B															
1.2 Retains one object when second object is obtained	B	B		B	B			B	B			B				B		
FS 1.2a Child retains object with one hand while acting on second object (e.g., child holds block while banging another block with other hand).																		
FS 1.2b Child retains one object while looking at second object.																		
2. Coordinates actions with objects to achieve new outcomes	B	B	B	B	B			B	B	B		B				B		
2.1 Tries different simple actions to achieve goal	B	B	B	B	B			B	B	B		B				B		
2.2 Uses simple actions on objects	B	B	B		B			B	B	B		B				B		

(page 32 of 42)

APPENDIX B: AEPS-3 SKILLS MATRIX

Cognitive (*continued*)

AEPS-3 Test Item

AEPS-3 Test Item	Active & Outdoor Play	Arrival & Departure	Art	Bath Time	Block Play	Circle Time	Diapering, Toileting, & Handwashing	Dramatic Play	Dressing	Field Trips	Math	Meals & Snacks	Music & Movement	Nap & Sleep	Science	Sensory	Technology	Writing
3. Solves problems using multiple strategies (RS 19)	R		R	R	R	R		R			R	R	R		R	R		R
3.1 Evaluates common solutions to solve problems or reach goals					G	G	G	G	G		G	G	G		G			
FS3.1a Child solves common problems (e.g., child pulls stool to cabinet to reach items on higher shelf).																		
FS3.1b Child suggests acceptable solutions to problems (e.g., when adult says she is cold, child offers, "We could turn up the heat").																		
FS3.1c Child uses adult to assist with solving common problem (e.g., child hands container to adult to help open it).																		
FS3.1d Child uses more than one strategy in attempt to solve common problem (e.g., child tugs on mother's pants to get attention, mother doesn't respond, child cries).																		
FS3.1e Child repeats same strategy to attempt to solve common problem (e.g., child tugs on mother's pants to get attention, mother doesn't respond, child tugs again).																		
4. Draws plausible conclusions about events beyond personal experience (RS 20)	R				R	R		R							R	R		R
4.1 Draws conclusions about causes of events based on personal experience		G		G	G	G	G	G		G					G			
E. Scientific Discovery																		
1. Expands simple observations and explorations into further inquiry (RS 21)	G	G		G	G	G				G					G	G		
1.1 Uses simple tools to gather information	G	G								G					G	G		
1.2 Uses senses to explore	B	B	B	B	B	B		B	B	B	B	B	B		B	B		B

APPENDIX B: AEPS-3 SKILLS MATRIX

Cognitive (continued)

AEPS-3 Test Item

AEPS-3 Curriculum Routine/Activity

AEPS-3 Test Item	Active & Outdoor Play	Arrival & Departure	Art	Bath Time	Block Play	Circle Time	Diapering, Toileting, & Handwashing	Dramatic Play	Dressing	Field Trips	Math	Meals & Snacks	Music & Movement	Nap & Sleep	Science	Sensory	Technology	Writing
2. Anticipates outcome of investigation (RS 22)																		
2.1 Generates specific questions for investigation	G	G								G					G			
2.2 Demonstrates knowledge about natural happenings				G		G				G		G			G			
2.3 Makes observations	B	B	B	B	B	B		B		B	B	B	B		G	B		B
3. Investigates to test hypotheses (RS 23)																		
3.1 Draws on prior knowledge to guide investigations					G					G					G			
3.2 Manipulates materials to cause change	G		G		G			R		G	G		G		G	G		G
4. Transfers knowledge (RS 24)																		
4.1 Communicates results of investigations	R	R	R	R	R	R				R	R		R		R	R	R	R
4.2 Demonstrates knowledge of properties of change resulting from investigations			R	R	R					R	R				R	R	R	
4.3 Shows awareness that manipulation of materials or processes prompted change in those materials or processes			R	R	R					R					R			

(page 34 of 42)

APPENDIX B: AEPS-3 SKILLS MATRIX

Literacy

AEPS-3 Curriculum Routine/Activity

AEPS-3 Test Item	Writing	Technology	Sensory	Science	Nap & Sleep	Music & Movement	Meals & Snacks	Math	Field Trips	Dressing	Dramatic Play	Diapering, Toileting, & Handwashing	Circle Time	Block Play	Bath Time	Art	Arrival & Departure	Active & Outdoor Play
A. Awareness of Print Concepts																		
1. Participates in shared group reading		G	G	G					G				G					
1.1 Participates in shared one-on-one reading	B		B		B				B		B		B		B			
FS 1.1a Child demonstrates functional use of reading materials while looking at picture books.																		
FS 1.1b Child orally fills in or completes familiar text while looking at picture books.																		
FS 1.1c Child indicates awareness that familiar text is left out or skipped over while looking at picture books.																		
FS 1.1d Child points to objects and answers questions while looking at picture books.																		
FS 1.1e Child responds to request to sit and read book with adult.																		
2. Demonstrates understanding that text is read in one direction and from top to bottom of page		G	G	G	G			G	G		G	G	G		G			
2.1 Turns pages of book from beginning toward end		G	G	G	G			G	G		G	G	G		G			
FS 2.1a Child attempts to turn pages.																		
2.2 Holds book or other printed material with pictures correctly oriented		G	G	G	G			G	G		G	G	G		G			
FS 2.2a Child holds books or other printed materials with or without pictures using both hands. Book does not need to be correctly oriented.																		
3. Recognizes print words for common or familiar people, objects, or pictures	R	R	R	R	R		R	R	R		R	R	R	R	R	R	R	
3.1 Recognizes own first name in print	R	R	R	R	R		G	R	G		G	R	G	R	R	G	G	G
3.2 Recognizes common signs and logos	G	G	G	G	G		G	G	G		G	G	G	G	G	G	G	G
B. Phonological Awareness																		
1. Produces rhyming words given oral prompt ▸ RS 25						R							R					
FS 1a Child produces some rhyming words in familiar rhymes.																		

APPENDIX B: AEPS-3 SKILLS MATRIX

Literacy (continued)

AEPS-3 Test Item	Active & Outdoor Play	Arrival & Departure	Art	Bath Time	Block Play	Circle Time	Diapering, Toileting, & Handwashing	Dramatic Play	Dressing	Field Trips	Math	Meals & Snacks	Music & Movement	Nap & Sleep	Science	Sensory	Technology	Writing
1.1 Identifies rhyming words						R							R					
FS 1.1a Child repeats simple nursery rhymes.																		
FS 1.1b Child says nursery rhymes along with familiar adult.																		
1.2 Participates in repetitive verbal play	G	G		G	G	G	G	G	G	G	G	G						
FS 1.2a Child indicates interest in hearing or repeating nursery rhymes.																		
2. Segments compound words into component words [RS 26]						R							R	R			R	
2.1 Blends two simple words into compound words						R							R					
2.2 Claps for words in sentences						R							R					
3. Segments syllables of two- and three-syllable words [RS 27]						R							R	R			R	
3.1 Blends syllables into two- and three-syllable words						R							R					
3.2 Claps for each syllable in two- and three-syllable words						R							R					
4. Segments CVC words into individual sounds [RS 28]						R							R	R			R	
4.1 Blends separate CVC sounds into simple words													R	R				
4.2 Identifies middle sounds in CVC words													R	R			R	
4.3 Identifies last sounds in CVC words						R							R	R			R	
4.4 Identifies beginning sounds in CVC words						R							R	R			R	
4.5 Produces words that begin with specified sound						R							R					

APPENDIX B: AEPS-3 SKILLS MATRIX

Literacy (continued)

AEPS-3 Test Item

AEPS-3 Curriculum Routine/Activity

AEPS-3 Test Item	Active & Outdoor Play	Arrival & Departure	Art	Bath Time	Block Play	Circle Time	Diapering, Toileting, & Handwashing	Dramatic Play	Dressing	Field Trips	Math	Meals & Snacks	Music & Movement	Nap & Sleep	Science	Sensory	Technology	Writing
C. Alphabet Knowledge																		
1. Names all uppercase and lowercase letters of alphabet [RS 29]	R	R		R	R	R	R	R	R	R		R	R				R	R
1.1 Matches frequently occurring lowercase letters with uppercase counterparts			R	R	R	R	R	R	R								R	R
1.2 Names 12 frequently occurring letters	R	R		R	R	R	R	R	R	R		R		R			R	R
1.3 Recognizes five frequently occurring letters not in first name			R			R		R		R					R			
1.4 Names letters in own first name	R	R	R	R	R	R	R	R	R	R		R		R	R		R	R
1.5 Recognizes three letters in own first name	R	R	R	R	R			R	R	R		R		R			R	R
2. Reads simple CVC and sight word text [RS 30]	R	R		R		R			R	R		R	R	R			R	
2.1 Sounds out CVC words	R	R		R					R	R			R	R				
2.2 Reads frequently occurring sight words	R	R		R						R	R	R	R	R	R		R	
FS 2.2a Child recognizes own name in print.				R	R							R	R	R			R	
2.3 Produces correct sounds for 20 letters of alphabet				R	R								R					
2.4 Produces correct sounds for six letters of alphabet				R	R								R					
D. Vocabulary and Story Comprehension																		
1. Demonstrates understanding that pictures represent text				G		G		G		G				G	G		G	G
1.1 Labels familiar people, actions, objects, and events in picture books				G		G		G		G				G	G	G	G	G
1.2 Locates familiar objects, people, events, and actions in picture books				G		G		G		G				G	G	G	G	
FS 1.2a Child locates common actions and events in familiar books or pictures.																		
FS 1.2b Child locates common objects and people in familiar books or pictures.											G							
1.3 Matches pictures to actual objects, people, or actions			G			G										G	G	

Assessment, Evaluation, and Programming System for Infants and Children, Third Edition (AEPS®-3), by Bricker, Dionne, Grisham, Johnson, Macy, Slentz, & Waddell. © 2022 Brookes Publishing Co. All rights reserved.

APPENDIX B: AEPS-3 SKILLS MATRIX

Literacy (continued)

AEPS-3 Test Item

AEPS-3 Curriculum Routine/Activity

AEPS-3 Test Item	Active & Outdoor Play	Arrival & Departure	Art	Bath Time	Block Play	Circle Time	Diapering, Toileting, & Handwashing	Dramatic Play	Dressing	Field Trips	Math	Meals & Snacks	Music & Movement	Nap & Sleep	Science	Sensory	Technology	Writing
2. Retells simple story **(RS 31)**			G	G		G				G				G	G		G	
2.1 Makes predictions about what will happen next in story						G				G				G	G		G	
2.2 Answers and asks questions related to story						G				G				G	G		G	
FS 2.2a Child makes comments related to story while looking at book (e.g., child points to lion in book and says "I went to the zoo").																		
2.3 Tells story associated with series of pictures			G			G				G				G	G		G	
3. Demonstrates understanding of abstract story vocabulary **(RS 32)**			G R			G R		G R		G R					G R		G R	
3.1 Demonstrates understanding of key vocabulary in picture books						G R				G R							G R	
3.2 Demonstrates understanding of title, author, and illustrator				R		G R				G				R	G R		G	
3.3 Demonstrates understanding of vocabulary associated with early literacy concepts						G				G				G	G		G	
E. Writing																		
1. "Reads" back own dictation to label or caption picture **(RS 33)**			R	R				R		G					R		R	R
1.1 Dictates description of drawing			R	G						R					G			G
1.2 Verbally labels representational drawings			G R	G R						G R					G R			G R

APPENDIX B: AEPS-3 SKILLS MATRIX

Literacy (continued)

AEPS-3 Test Item

AEPS-3 Curriculum Routine/Activity

AEPS-3 Test Item	Writing	Technology	Sensory	Science	Nap & Sleep	Music & Movement	Meals & Snacks	Math	Field Trips	Dressing	Dramatic Play	Diapering, Toileting, & Handwashing	Circle Time	Block Play	Bath Time	Art	Arrival & Departure	Active & Outdoor Play
1.3 Verbally labels nonrepresentational drawings	G			G					G						G	G		G
2. Writes and draws for a variety of purposes [RS 34]	R	R		R					R		R				R	R	R	R
2.1 Makes representational drawings	R	G		R							G				G	G		G
3. Writes words using conventional spelling	G	R		G				R	R		R				R	R	R	R
3.1 Writes using developmental spelling	R	R		R				R	R		R				R	R	R	R
3.2 Prints first name	R	R		R					R		R				R	R	R	R
FS 3.2a Child prints three letters.																		
3.3 Copies entire first name	R	R		R					R		R				R	R	R	
FS 3.3a Child copies three letters.																		
FS 3.3b Child copies complex shapes.																		
FS 3.3c Child copies simple shapes.																		
3.4 Writes using "scribble writing"	R	R		R												R	R	R

APPENDIX B: AEPS-3 SKILLS MATRIX

Math

AEPS-3 Curriculum Routine/Activity

A. Counting

AEPS-3 Test Item	Active & Outdoor Play	Arrival & Departure	Art	Bath Time	Block Play	Circle Time	Diapering, Toileting, & Handwashing	Dramatic Play	Dressing	Field Trips	Math	Meals & Snacks	Music & Movement	Nap & Sleep	Science	Sensory	Technology	Writing
1. Counts out 3 items	G	G	G	G	G	G	G	G	G	G	G	G		G	G	G	G	G
1.1 Counts 3 items to determine "How many?"	G	G	G	G	G	G	G	G	G	G	G	G		G	G	G	G	G
FS 1.1a Child demonstrates one-to-one correspondence by assigning one of two objects to another person and keeping other object (e.g., child gives one of two daisies to father, keeps other daisy).																		
FS 1.1b Child demonstrates concept of one (e.g., when told child can have one cookie, child takes only one).																		
1.2 Recites numbers 1–3	B	B	B	B	B	B	B	B	B	B	B	B	B	B		B		B
2. Counts out 10 items	R	R	R	R	R	R		R	R	R	R	R		R	R	R	R	R
2.1 Counts 10 items to determine "How many?"	R	R	R	R	R	R	R	R	R	R	R	R	R	R	R	R	R	R
2.2 Recites numbers 1–10	R	R	R		R	G	G	G	G		G			R	R	R	R	R
3. Counts out 20 items	R	R	R	R	R	R	R	R		R	R	R	R	R	R	R	R	R
3.1 Counts 20 items to determine "How many?"	R	R	R	R	R	R	R	R	R	R	R	R	R	R	R	R	R	R
3.2 Recites numbers 1–20	R	R	R	R	R	R		R		R	R	R		R	R	R	R	R
4. Skip counts by tens to 100	R	R	R	R	R	R			R	R	R	R		R	R	R	R	R
4.1 Recites numbers 31–100	R	R	R	R	R	R	R			R	R	R		R	R	R	R	R
4.2 Recites numbers 1–30	R	R	R	R	R	R			R	R	R	R		R	R	R	R	R

B. Quantitative Relations

AEPS-3 Test Item	Active & Outdoor Play	Arrival & Departure	Art	Bath Time	Block Play	Circle Time	Diapering, Toileting, & Handwashing	Dramatic Play	Dressing	Field Trips	Math	Meals & Snacks	Music & Movement	Nap & Sleep	Science	Sensory	Technology	Writing
1. Compares items in sets to 5 by counting					G			G		G	G	G			G	G	G	
1.1 Compares items in sets to 5 by matching					G			G		G	G				G	G	G	

APPENDIX B: AEPS-3 SKILLS MATRIX

Math (continued)

AEPS-3 Test Item	Writing	Technology	Sensory	Science	Nap & Sleep	Music & Movement	Meals & Snacks	Math	Field Trips	Dressing	Dramatic Play	Diapering, Toileting, & Handwashing	Circle Time	Block Play	Bath Time	Art	Arrival & Departure	Active & Outdoor Play
1.2 Creates equivalent sets of 5 items		G	G	G			G	G	G		G		G	G		G	G	
1.3 Uses quantity comparison words FS 1.3a Child demonstrates understanding of quantity words (e.g., child points to person at table who has more).	G		G	G				G	G	G	G		G	G		G		
2. Compares items in sets of 6 to 10 by counting		R	R	R				R			R		R	R	R	R	R	R
2.1 Compares items in sets of 6 to 10 by matching		R	R	R				R			R			R	R	R	R	R
2.2 Creates equivalent sets of 10 items		R	R	R				R			R			R		R		R
3. Compares items in sets of 11 to 20 by counting RS 35		R	R	R				R			R		R	R	R		R	R
3.1 Compares items in sets of 11 to 20 by matching		R	R	R				R			R			R		R		R
3.2 Compares items in sets of 11 to 20 by visual examination		R	R	R				R			R		R	R	R	R		R
C. Reading and Writing Numbers																		
1. Reads and writes numerals for quantities to 5 RS 36	R	R	R	R	R		R	R	R		R		R	R	R	R	R	R
1.1 Demonstrates understanding of mathematical meaning of written numerals 1–5	R	R	R	R	R		R	R	R		R		R	R	R	R	R	R
1.2 Labels numerals 1–5	R	R	R	R			R	R	R		R		R	R		R	R	R
2. Reads and writes numerals for quantities 6–10 RS 37	R	R	R	R	R		R	R	R		R		R	R	R	R	R	R
2.1 Demonstrates understanding of mathematical meaning of written numerals 6–10	R	R	R	R			R	R	R		R		R	R	R	R	R	R
2.2 Labels numerals 6–10	R	R	R	R	R		R	R	R		R		R	R		R		R
3. Reads and writes numerals for quantities 11–20 RS 38	R	R	R	R	R		R	R	R		R		R	R		R	R	R
3.1 Demonstrates understanding of mathematical meaning of written numerals 11–20	R	R	R	R			R	R	R		R		R	R		R		R
3.2 Labels numerals 11–20	R	R	R	R			R		R		R			R		R	R	R

APPENDIX B: AEPS-3 SKILLS MATRIX

Math *(continued)*

AEPS-3 Test Item

D. Addition and Subtraction

AEPS-3 Test Item	Active & Outdoor Play	Arrival & Departure	Art	Bath Time	Block Play	Circle Time	Diapering, Toileting, & Handwashing	Dramatic Play	Dressing	Field Trips	Math	Meals & Snacks	Music & Movement	Nap & Sleep	Science	Sensory	Technology	Writing
1. Reads and writes symbols for addition (+) and equals (=) *(RS 39)*				R							R				R		R	R
1.1 Solves picture or object addition problems using shortcut sum strategy			R	R							R				R		R	R
1.2 Counts forward to 10	R		R	R	R	R	R	R	R	R	R	R		R	R	R	R	R
1.3 Solves picture or object problems using count all strategy			R	R							R				R		R	R
1.4 Says number after 1–10	R		R	R	R	R	R			R	R	R	R	R	R	R	R	R
1.5 Demonstrates understanding of concept of addition			R	R	R	R		R			R	R		R	R	R	R	R
2. Reads and writes symbols for subtraction (−) and equals (=) *(RS 40)*	R			R	R	R		R			R				R		R	R
2.1 Solves picture or object subtraction problems with set of 10 or less	R		R	R			R				R			R	R	R	R	R
2.2 Says number before 2–10			R	R	R	R				R	R	R		R	R	R	R	R
2.3 Demonstrates understanding of concept of subtraction			R	R	R	R		R		R	R	R		R	R	R	R	R

Index

Page numbers followed by *f* and *t* indicate figures and tables, respectively.

Is your aeps3 system complete?

A highly effective and efficient linked system, **Assessment, Evaluation, and Programming System for Infants and Children, Third Edition (AEPS®-3)** gives your early childhood program the **most accurate, useful child data** and a **proven way to turn data into action** across everything you do, from goal setting to teaching to progress monitoring. The complete system includes:

AEPS®-3 User's Guide (Volume 1)

Comprehensive and reader-friendly, this User's Guide gives early childhood professionals the practical knowledge they need to use AEPS-3 accurately and effectively.

US$50.00 • Stock #: BA-55194 • ISBN 978-1-68125-519-4

AEPS®-3 Assessment (Volume 2)

The assessment volume covers test items and criteria; administration and scoring guidelines; and use of assessment activities, Ready-Set assessment, and family materials.

US$100.00 • Stock #: BA-55200 • ISBN 978-1-68125-520-0

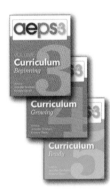

AEPS®-3 Curriculum

For use after the AEPS-3 Test, the AEPS-3 Curriculum is an activity-based, multitiered curriculum that helps professionals support every child's development with differentiated instruction.

Beginning (Volume 3)

US$50.00 • Stock #: BA-55217 • ISBN 978-1-68125-521-7

Growing (Volume 4)

US$50.00 • Stock #: BA-55224 • ISBN 978-1-68125-522-4

Ready (Volume 5)

US$50.00 • Stock #: BA-55231 • ISBN 978-1-68125-523-1

AEPS®-3 Forms USB

USB includes printable PDFs of AEPS-3 forms (in English and Spanish), plus handouts for families (in English and Spanish), Assessment Activities (English only), and more.

US$299.00 • Stock #: BA-55248 • ISBN 978-1-68125-524-8

Forms also available in paper format; see www.aepsinteractive.com

---

AEPSi Online System

Turn your data into action with the intuitive, user-friendly AEPSi online system. With powerful scoring and reporting options, customized data collection forms, and a family login for communication, AEPSi will help you save time and support real progress for every child.

Discover the benefits of AEPSi with a demo or free trial! Visit www.aepsinteractive.com

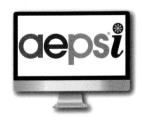

COMPLETE YOUR SYSTEM TODAY!

Call 1-800-638-3775   **Online https://aepsinteractive.com**

Your listcode is BA

Prices subject to change